Equine Endoscopy

EQUINE ENDOSCOPY

EDITED BY

JOSIE L. TRAUB-DARGATZ, D.V.M., M.S.

Associate Professor of Medicine, Department of Clinical Sciences
Colorado State University
College of Veterinary Medicine and Biomedical Sciences
Fort Collins, Colorado

CHRISTOPHER M. BROWN, B.Sc., B.V.Sc., Ph.D.,
M.R.C.V.S.

Professor, Department of Large Animal Clinical Sciences
Michigan State University
College of Veterinary Medicine
East Lansing, Michigan

with 23 black and white and 244 four-color illustrations

THE C. V. MOSBY COMPANY

ST. LOUIS • BALTIMORE • PHILADELPHIA • TORONTO   1990

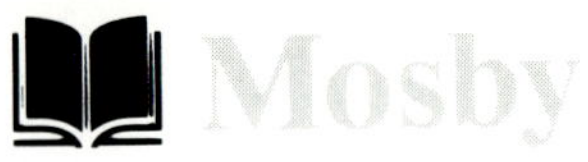

Editor: Robert W. Reinhardt
Assistant Editor: Melba Steube
Project Manager: Mark Spann
Production Editor: Daniel J. Johnson
Designer: Liz Fett

Library of Congress Cataloging-in-Publication Data

Equine endoscopy / edited by Josie L. Traub-Dargatz and Christopher M.
    Brown.
            p.   cm.
        Includes index
        ISBN 0-8016-3240-4
        1. Horses—Diseases—Diagnosis.   2. Veterinary endoscopy.
    I. Traub-Dargatz, Josie L.   II. Brown, Christopher M.
        [DNLM: 1. Endoscopy—veterinary.   2. Horse Diseases—diagnosis.
    SF 951 E635]
    SF951.E55   1990
    636.1.′089607545—dc20
    DNLM/DLC
    for Library of Congress   89-13527
                                                                        CIP

Printed in the United States of America

The C. V. Mosby Company
11830 Westline Industrial Drive, St. Louis, Missouri 63146

C/W/W 9 8 7 6 5 4 3 2 1

CONTRIBUTORS

PETER J. W. ADAMSON,
B.Sc., B.V.M.S.

Visiting Fellow, Veterinary Clinical
  Studies
Murdoch University Veterinary School
Murdoch, Western Australia;
Private Practitioner, Baldivis Veterinary
  Hospital
Baldivis, Western Australia, Australia

JOSEPH J. BERTONE,
D.V.M., M.S.

Assistant Professor, Department of
  Veterinary Clinical Sciences
The Ohio State University College of
  Veterinary Medicine
Columbus, Ohio

CARLA L. CARLETON,
D.V.M., M.S.

Associate Professor, Department of
  Large Animal Clinical Sciences
Michigan State University
College of Veterinary Medicine
East Lansing, Michigan

JOHN P. CARON, D.V.M., M.V.Sc.

Assistant Professor, Department of
  Large Animal Clinical Sciences
Michigan State University
College of Veterinary Medicine
East Lansing, Michigan

BENJAMIN J. DARIEN,
D.V.M., M.S.

Assistant Professor, Department of
  Large Animal Medicine
Oregon State University
College of Veterinary Medicine
Corvallis, Oregon

FREDERIK J. DERKSEN,
D.V.M., Ph.D.

Professor, Department of Large Animal
  Clinical Sciences
Michigan State University
College of Veterinary Medicine
East Lansing, Michigan

A. TED FISCHER, JR.,
D.V.M.

Private Practitioner
Chino Valley Equine Hospital
Chino, California

PETER F. HAYNES, D.V.M., M.S.

Professor, Department of Veterinary
  Clinical Sciences
Louisiana State University
School of Veterinary Medicine
Baton Rouge, Louisiana

ANN M. LAMAR, L.V.T.

Veterinary Technician II
Veterinary Clinical Center
Michigan State University
College of Veterinary Medicine
East Lansing, Michigan

MICHAEL J. MURRAY,
D.V.M., M.S.

Assistant Professor, Department of
  Large Animal Clinical Sciences
Virginia–Maryland Regional College of
  Veterinary Medicine, Virginia Tech,
Blacksburg; and Marion duPont Scott
  Equine Medical Center
Leesburg, Virginia

FRANK A. NICKELS,
D.V.M., M.S.

Associate Professor, Department of
  Large Animal Clinical Sciences
Michigan State University
College of Veterinary Medicine
East Lansing, Michigan

JOHN A. STICK, D.V.M.

Professor, Department of Large Animal
  Clinical Sciences
Michigan State University
College of Veterinary Medicine
East Lansing, Michigan

KENNETH E. SULLINS,
D.V.M., M.S.

Associate Professor, Department of
  Large Animal Clinical Sciences
Virginia-Maryland Regional College of
  Veterinary Medicine, Virginia Tech
Blacksburg; and Marion duPont Scott
  Equine Medical Center
Leesburg, Virginia

WALTER R. THRELFALL,
D.V.M., M.S., Ph.D.

Professor, Department of Veterinary
  Clinical Sciences
The Ohio State University
College of Veterinary Medicine
Columbus, Ohio

ERIC P. TULLENERS, D.V.M.

Assistant Professor, Department of
  Clinical Studies
New Bolton Center
University of Pennsylvania
School of Veterinary Medicine
Kennett Square, Pennsylvania

*To all the patients
who helped us to learn the contents
of this text*

PREFACE

Our purpose in assembling this text was four-fold:

- To compile in a single text, with an easy-to-use format, the basics of equine endoscopy.
- To instruct the reader on how to do endoscopy of various locations in the body of the horse.
- To aid the reader in selection of appropriate endoscopic equipment for the task at hand.
- To illustrate abnormal endoscopic findings and to cover indications for endoscopy of a given site in the horse.

We intended only to show the diagnostic value of the endoscope, not to discuss the management of the abnormal conditions detected by endoscopy as this information can be found in a number of other resources in the veterinary literature. It is our hope that the clinician's diagnostic skills learned through this work might enhance the quality and satisfaction of equine practice for both the student and the practitioner.

JOSIE L. TRAUB-DARGATZ
CHRISTOPHER M. BROWN

CONTENTS

Chapter 1

STANDARD FIBEROPTIC EQUIPMENT AND ITS CARE

ANN M. LAMAR

FIBEROPTIC PRINCIPLES

Fiberoptic endoscopy is a system used to transmit light and images through long thin fibers of optical glass. These glass fibers transmit light only when the adjacent medium has a lower refractive index. Therefore, each glass fiber is coated with a thin layer of lower refractive index glass (cladding glass), which ensures that the majority of light entering the fiber will reach the distal end rather than leak through to adjacent objects. Because a single fiber cannot transmit an image (the pattern made by the transmitted light and color), thousands of fibers are bundled together.

The modern endoscope has two types of fiber bundles — the image guide (IG) bundle and the light guide (LG) bundle. Each endoscope has only one IG bundle, which consists of 5000 to 40,000 individual fibers that are arranged coherently. Each fiber must occupy the same position at the proximal end as it does in the distal end or the image will be distorted. When one of the fibers breaks, a black dot appears in the image (Fig. 1-1) because light is no longer being transmitted by that fiber. The number of fibers in the IG bundle varies greatly, depending on the size and type of endoscope. Larger endoscopes, such as the colonoscope, have larger IG bundles that produce images of superior quality.

The LG bundle transmits light from the light source to the distal end of the endoscope. Because they do not have to transmit an im-

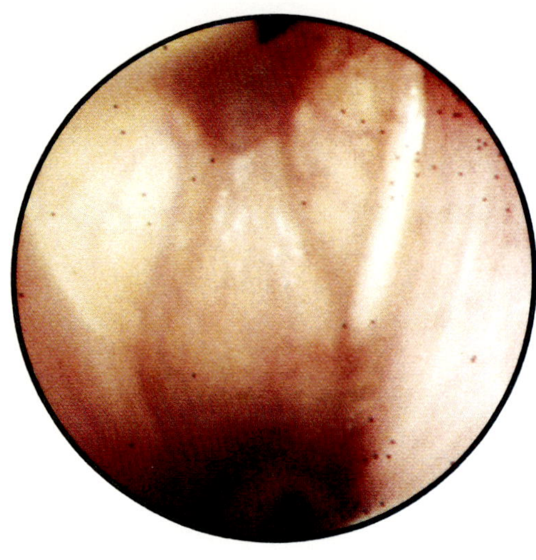

FIG. 1-1 The black dots in this photograph represent broken fibers.

age, these fibers are arranged randomly (incoherently) and each fiber is larger and thicker and therefore more efficient at transmitting light. Except for the very small models, many endoscopes contain two LG bundles.

In addition to the fiber bundle system, each endoscope contains three lens systems: (1) the light guide lens system (illumination lens), which distributes light from the LG bundle into wide angle illumination (2) the objective lens system, which focuses the image onto the IG bundle and (3) the ocular lens system, which is located in the control head and acts as a magnifying glass so that the observer can see the image taken into the IG bundle.

ENDOSCOPIC CONSTRUCTION

The external parts of the endoscope are identified in Fig. 1-2.

Distal tip

The typical endoscope, as seen in Fig. 1-3, houses the objective lens of the image guide bundle, the illumination lenses of the light guide bundles, the distal channel opening for suction and passage of endoscopic accessories, and the air/water channel nozzle. Some endoscopes have a detachable rubber hood that keeps the objective lens away from the mucosa.

Bending section

The majority of flexible endoscopes have in their design a bending section that allows the distal end to turn right, left, up, or down, greatly increasing the field of view (Fig. 1-4). The degree of deflection varies among types of endoscopes. The current design of the

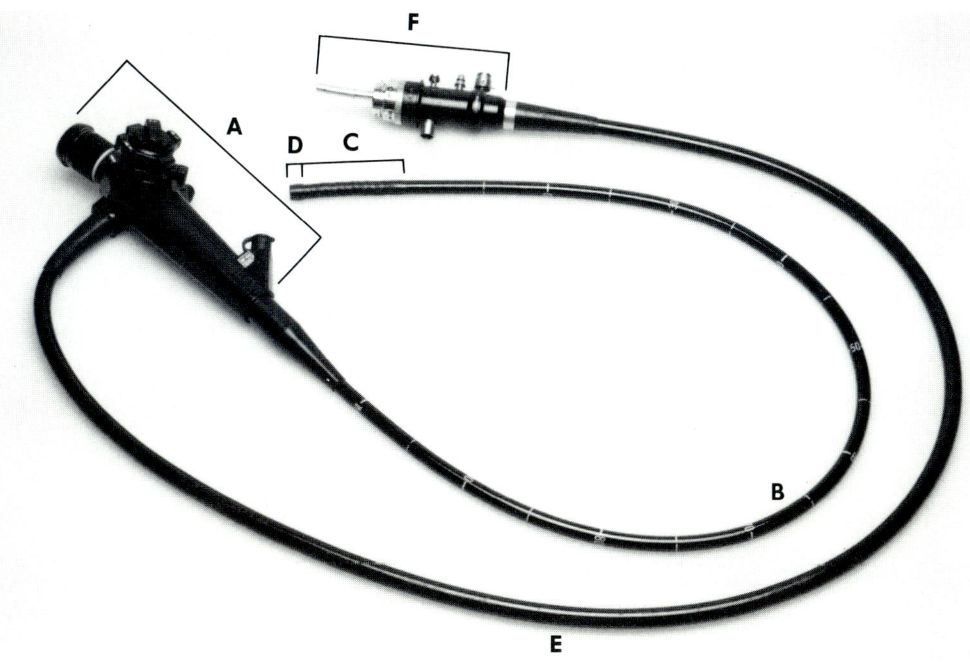

FIG. 1-2 A Fiberoptic endoscope. *A,* Control section; *B,* insertion tube; *C,* bending section; *D,* distal tip; *E,* universal cord; *F,* light guide connector.

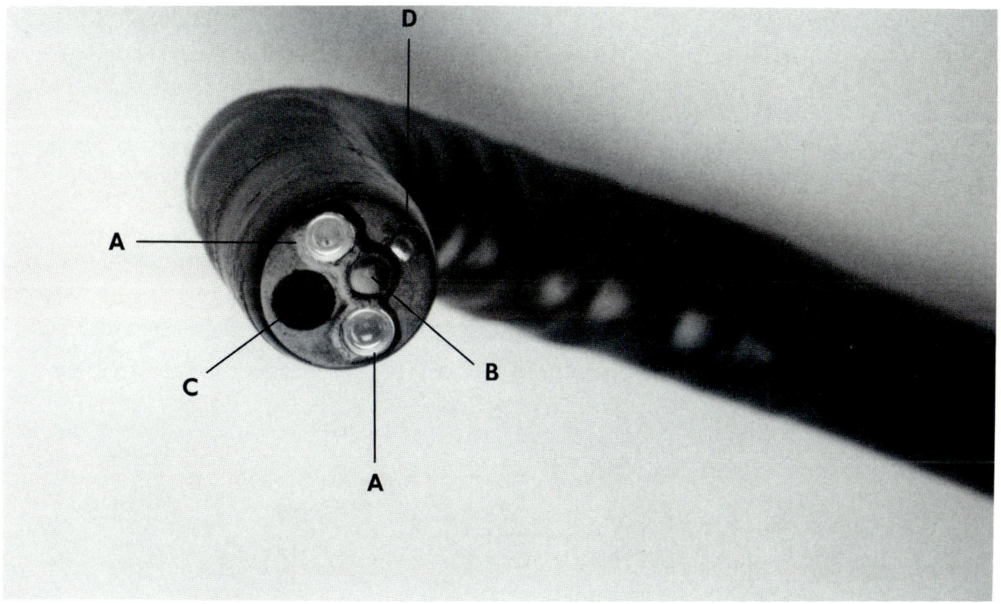

FIG. 1-3 End view of the distal tip of the insertion tube. *A,* Illumination lenses of the light guide bundles; *B,* objective lens of the image guide bundle; *C,* accessory channel opening; *D,* air/water nozzle.

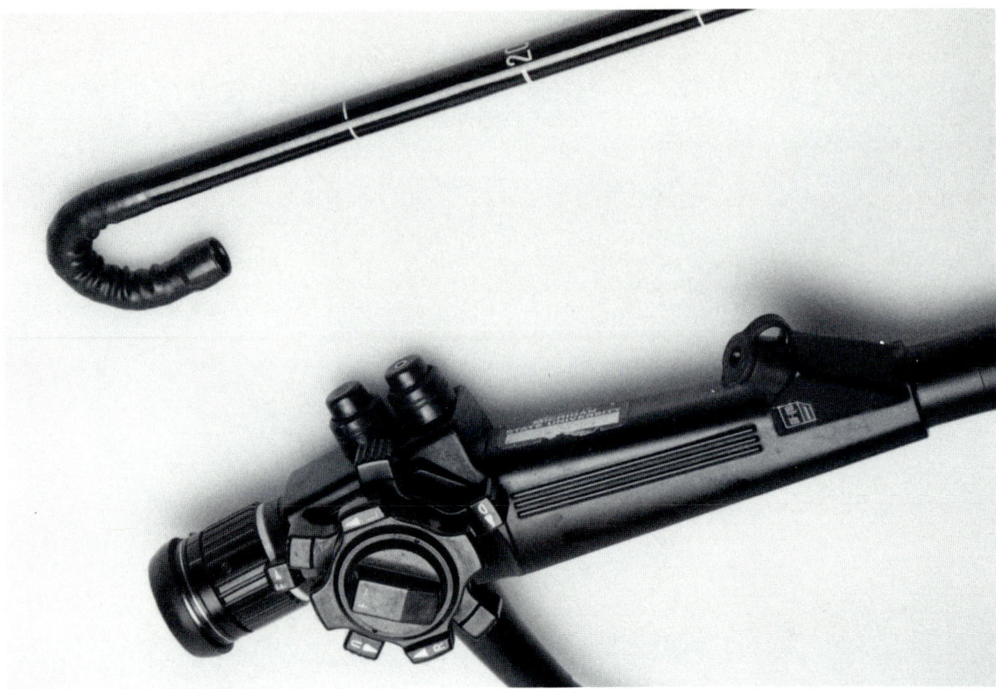

FIG. 1-4 Deflection of the bending section occurs in all planes in most fiberoptic endoscopes.

bending section includes a series of interlocking metal rings, each with four joints that allow deflection in any direction. Angulation control wires run the length of the insertion tube, from the metal rings to the controls on the control section. The controls are able to lock into position, enabling the endoscopist to release the control knob while maintaining the desired deflection.

Insertion tube

The insertion tube is flexible along its entire length, although flexibility decreases near the control section. Steel bands in a spiral pattern give the insertion tube its round shape and protect the delicate internal structures. A steel wire mesh covers the steel bands and helps prevent twisting and stretching of the insertion tube and its contents. The plastic covering of this portion of the endoscope is waterproof and able to withstand chemical agents, such as disinfectants and gastric acid.

Control section

The control section of the endoscope has undergone a great deal of change in design over the years, but the content has remained virtually the same. This section is designed to be held in the left hand. The index finger of the left hand operates the air/water and suction

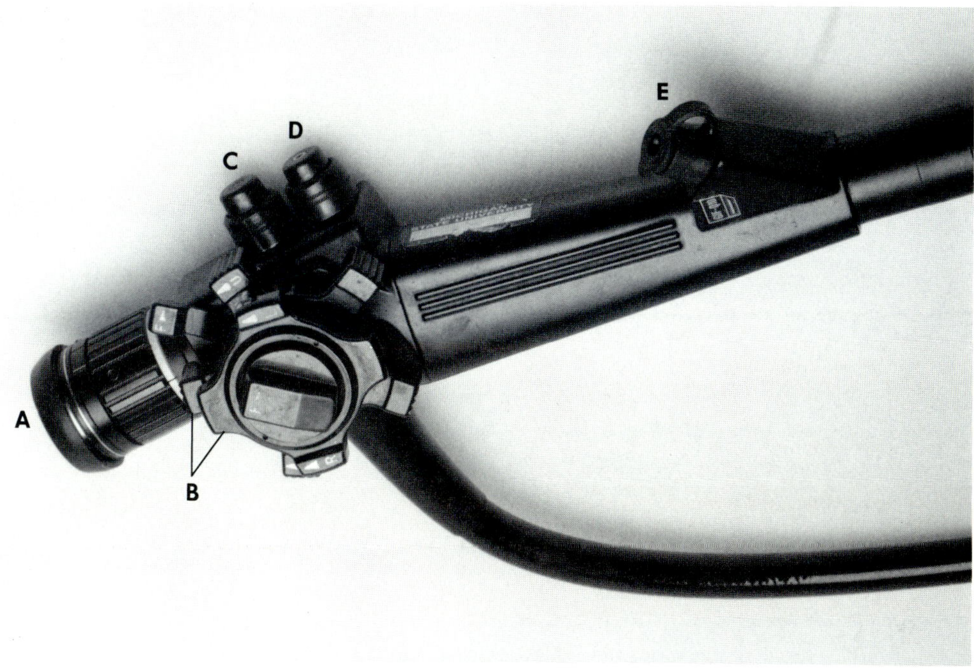

FIG. 1-5 The control section of the modern fiberoptic endoscope. *A,* Eye piece; *B,* deflection control knobs; *C,* suction valve; *D,* air/water valve; *E,* opening to accessory channel.

valves, and the thumb moves the up/down control knob. The right hand manipulates the insertion tube, passes accessories into the accessory channel, and turns the right/left control knob (Fig. 1-5).

Located within the control section are the air, water, and suction systems. The light source itself houses an air pump; air exits at the nozzle on the distal tip of the endoscope when the opening in the air/water valve is covered. Air is used to insufflate structures being examined, such as the esophagus, vagina, or uterus of a mare. It is also useful in blowing water off the objective lens after it has been rinsed to remove secretions. Water is flushed through the system from a water bottle attached to the light guide connector when the air/water valve is fully depressed.

A separate suction unit can be used to suction materials through the endoscope. Tubing from the suction unit can be attached to the endoscope at the light guide connector. Depressing the suction valve will aspirate fluid or air when the suction unit is operating.

Light guide connector

The universal cord attaches the control section of the endoscope to the light guide connector, which is inserted into the light source. The light guide connector has connections for the water bottle, suc-

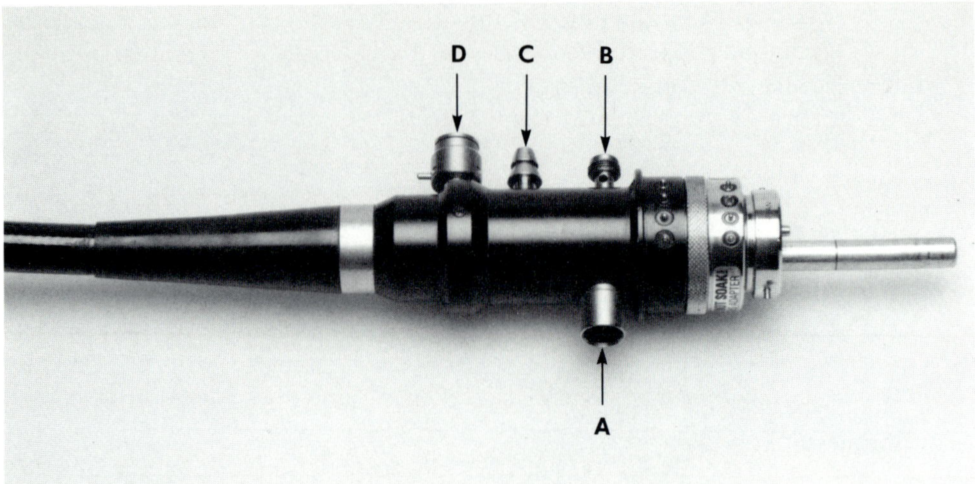

FIG. 1-6   The light guide connector has receptacles for the: *A,* Water bottle; *B,* electrosurgical safety cord; *C,* suction apparatus; *D,* venting cap for immersible models used during ethylene oxide sterilization.

tion apparatus, electrosurgical safety cord, CO_2 attachments, and a venting connector for immersible endoscopes used for ethylene oxide sterilization (Fig. 1-6).

ANCILLARY EQUIPMENT

Light sources

Endoscopic light sources available today range from the very simple to the complex. All are cold light sources, a major improvement over earlier light sources, which produced increased temperatures at the distal end. All have the ability to increase or decrease light intensity during the procedure, but the type of light used varies among light sources. Currently, the two types of light used are halogen and xenon. Xenon lamps produce a bluish-white light, similar to daylight, which is much brighter than the yellow halogen lamp. Although many halogen light sources are equipped with automatic exposure flashes for photography, only the higher-powered xenon light sources are suitable for video photography. The xenon light source and replacement lamp are substantially higher in price than the halogen counterpart, but the xenon lamp has a much longer life. Selection of the type of light to be used should be based on intended use and personal preference.

Another factor in light source selection is the availability of an air/water pump. Most light sources feature the option, but the very simple models do not.

Endoscopes and light sources produced by major manufacturers are often interchangeable. Some manufacturers provide adapters fitted to the light guide connector and/or light source, while others include a separate receptacle on the light source for other manufacturers' fiberoptic endoscopes.

Cameras

When selecting endoscopic equipment, it is very important to consider the desired options before making the final purchase. This is especially true when considering photography, where selecting the appropriate light source is essential. Proper illumination is the key to obtaining quality photographs. This is influenced somewhat by the size of the light guide bundles in the endoscope but more so by the light source. Xenon light sources are usually much brighter than halogen light sources. Both types offer a built in flash, and many provide automatic film exposure as well.

Once the light source is selected, the camera can be chosen. Each of the major endoscope manufacturers makes cameras specifically for the endoscope. These cameras produce high-quality still photographs and are fully automatic. Through electronic signals sent to the light source, they are able to adjust shutter speed, brightness, and flash duration. They also automatically compensate for distance of the object from the endoscope and image magnification and color. Many of these cameras use 110 cassette film.

A 35 mm single lens reflex (SLR) camera, with a special adapter that fits it to the endoscope eyepiece, may be used to take still photographs (Fig. 1-7). Major manufacturers provide adapters that adapt their endoscopes to cameras from a different manufacturer; for example, a Pentax endoscope can be adapted to fit an Olympus camera. Many adapters have electrical contacts that transmit information to the light source, which produces the flash and controls the film exposure (Fig. 1-8). Film for the 35 mm camera is selected according to the type of light source to be used. Tungsten film is required when using a halogen light source, while daylight film is used for systems with xenon light sources.

Also available are instant film cameras, which produce a print of the image within minutes. The film is manufactured by Polaroid and is available through several endoscope manufacturers. This camera also requires a special adapter to attach it to the endoscope eyepiece.

Video endoscopes have recently become available and are valuable for teaching and when documentation of endoscopic findings is desired. The video endoscope will be discussed in detail in Chapter 2.

Electrosurgical units

Electrosurgery, such as polypectomy and cauterization, can be done utilizing instruments that are passed through the endoscope acces-

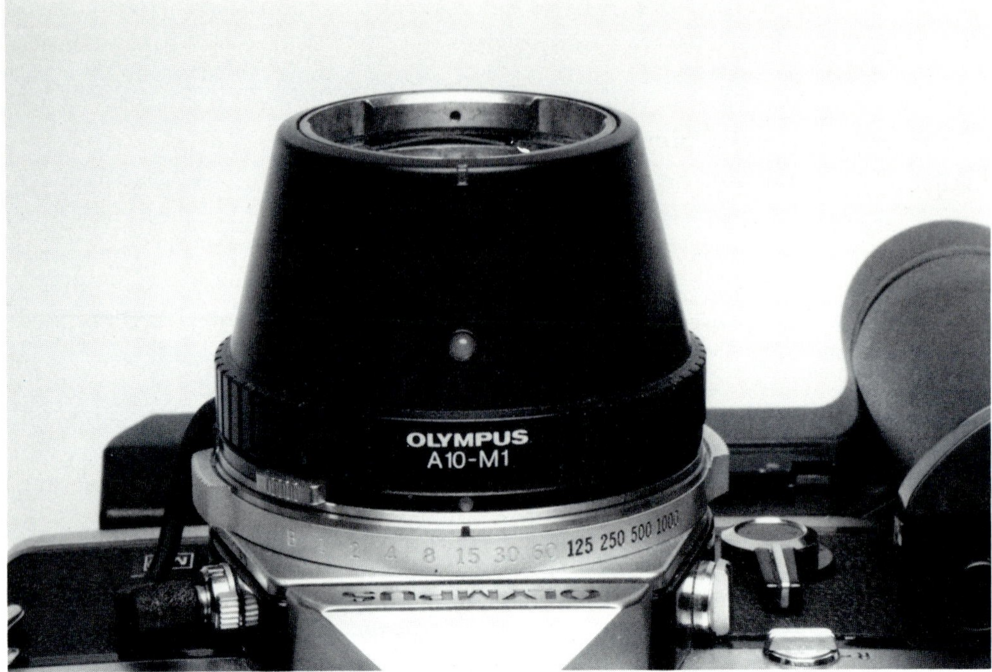

FIG. 1-7   35 mm SLR camera requiring special adapter to fit the eye piece of the endoscope.

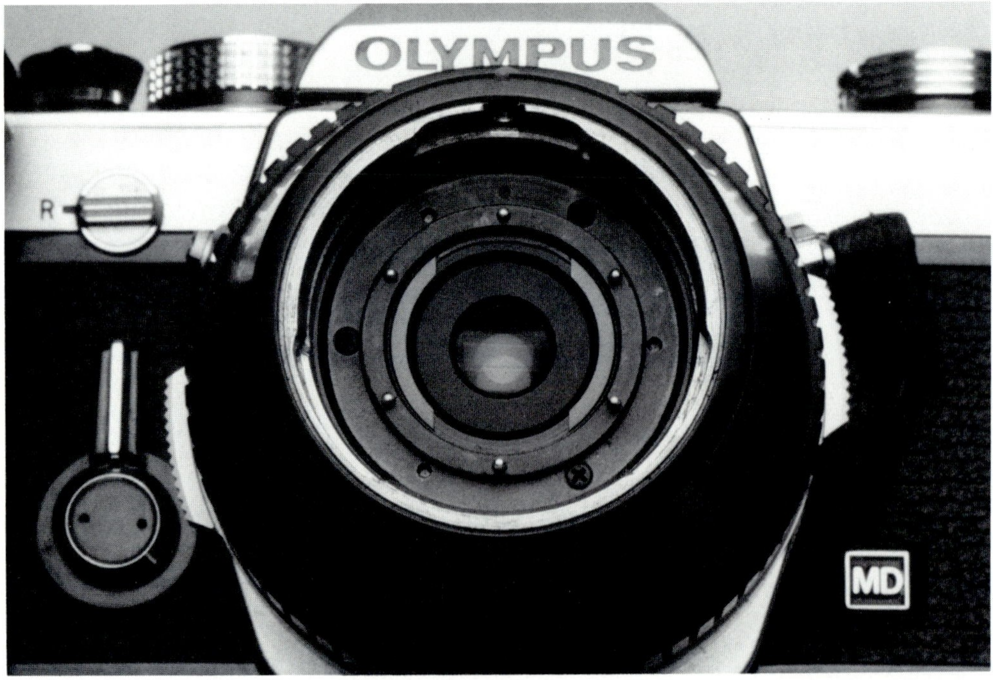

FIG. 1-8   Most camera adapters, like the one shown above, have electrical contacts that transmit information to the light source to produce a flash and control film exposure.

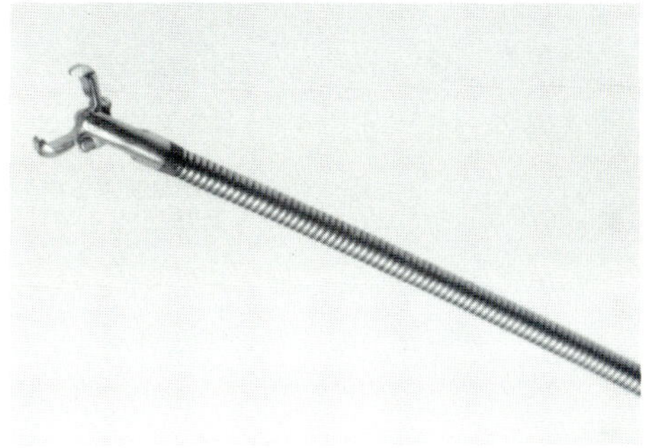

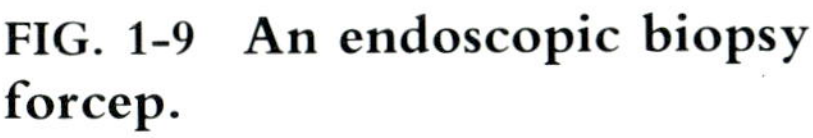
FIG. 1-9 **An endoscopic biopsy forcep.**

sory channel. These instruments receive power from the electrosurgical units to which they are attached. Electrosurgical units used for general surgical procedures can be adapted to receive instruments, but some endoscope manufacturers have designed their own units with endoscopic surgical procedures in mind; for example, units with built-in safety features to reduce the incidence of accidents during the procedure. Special features include a safety return cord that returns current leaks back to the unit; a built-in warning system for improper connections; and automatic shutdown if the returned current is excessive. Many units may also be used for general surgical procedures.

ENDOSCOPIC ACCESSORIES

Biopsy forceps are used when a small biopsy of an observable lesion is desired. Many different styles of biopsy instruments are available in various sizes and lengths to fit the many sizes and styles of endoscopes (Fig. 1-9). They include round or oval cups with or without needles, fenestrated cups, and alligator forceps.

Cytology brushes are used to retrieve specimens for cytologic examination. They are available in disposable and reusable styles. Brushes are also made to obtain microbiology samples using a unique double catheter system. A water soluble wax plug seals the outer catheter. When the instrument is positioned in the desired location, the plug is pushed out, a second catheter emerges, and the sterile brush is passed through it into the area to be sampled. This catheter is available from Mill-Rose Laboratories, Inc. Cytology brushes are made in several sizes and lengths corresponding to the type of endoscope used.

A double-catheter tracheal aspiration apparatus is currently being developed by Mill-Rose Laboratories, Inc. It operates much like the microbiology cytology brush. A small amount of sterile saline is injected through the sterile internal catheter and, by visualization, the resultant wash is aspirated. Since the sample is collected in a sterile

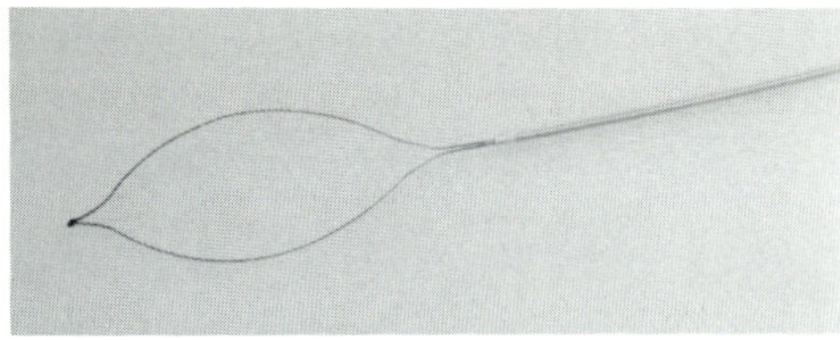

FIG. 1-10 A diathermic snare used for polypectomies.

manner, it can be submitted for microbiologic examination. When used properly, this system can replace the invasive transtracheal aspiration procedure with reliable results.

Cytology samples may also be obtained by using a non-sterile washing pipe. This pipe is a single, open tube that can be used to aspirate fluid and wash or treat a specific area of the upper respiratory or digestive system. Washing pipes are available in various sizes.

Grasping forceps or retrieval baskets, available in many styles and sizes, can be used to retrieve foreign bodies.

Electrosurgery can be done through the endoscope using various types of instruments. The coagulation electrode has a rounded end for localized coagulation. Polyps can be removed with diathermic snares (Fig. 1-10). Hot biopsy forceps may be used to obtain a biopsy and to control hemorrhage simultaneously. Each of these accessories is available in many sizes and styles to correspond to the endoscope being used.

HANDLING THE ENDOSCOPE

Pre-use inspection

Thoroughly examine the endoscope before each use. If there are cracks in the external surface, fluid may leak into the fiber bundle system and seriously damage the endoscope. Damage can be assessed quickly by looking into the endoscope and evaluating the clearness of the image. In the early stages, the image will appear foggy, and adjusting the eyepiece focusing apparatus will not alter it. If severe damage has occurred, the affected portion will be blackened or smeared, and thorough cleaning of the lens systems will not improve the image. If any of these abnormalities exists, do not use the endoscope.

Test the bending section of the insertion tube by manipulating the control knobs to ensure that deflection in all planes is present. Never manually bend the tip. If the bending section is not working properly, the cables may be stretched or broken and, therefore, will need repair before continued use.

Air/water, and suction valves should move easily and perform their desired functions. If they are not operating properly, examine all connections between the power source and the endoscope. If the endoscope is not seated securely into the power source, these functions are inhibited. If the water bottle is not filled or attached properly to the light guide connector, depressing the air/water valve will not produce air or water at the distal tip. If the connections are correct and these functions are not working, do not use the endoscope.

Evaluate the fiber bundle system frequently. This way proper or improper handling of the endoscope by those involved with its use can be monitored. With the light source on, focus the endoscope on a nearby object and count the number of black dots present. This number represents the number of broken fibers in the endoscope. If the broken fibers are scattered, the breakage is probably due to normal use, but if they are concentrated in one specific area, excessive bending or abuse has occurred.

Transportation

When performing an endoscopic examination inside a clinic, it is advantageous to store all equipment on a sturdy cart with wheels. If the patient reacts unfavorably to the examination, the equipment can be moved aside quickly and safely.

In an ambulatory practice, proper transportation of endoscopic equipment is essential. The endoscope should always be placed in its protective case, which has thick padding to keep the endoscope in one position and additional spaces for the water bottle, camera, and accessories. Table-top light sources are equipped with handles for transportation.

Another important factor to consider in an ambulatory practice is the effect of cold environmental conditions on the equipment. When the glass fibers become cold, they are very susceptible to breakage; therefore, the endoscope should be warmed as much as possible before use. This may be accomplished by keeping the equipment on the front seat of a heated vehicle.

Care throughout the examination

It goes without saying that in order to perform a good diagnostic examination, the patient must cooperate. Therefore, proper restraint is essential to protect not only the patient and personnel involved but also the endoscopic equipment. If the animal is not restrained in examination stocks, make certain that the equipment is not placed directly in front of or next to the patient. If there is no alternative but to place it close to the patient, provide a means of moving it out of the way quickly, if necessary.

Lubricating the distal end of the insertion tube will facilitate placement of the endoscope into the desired location. Do this by applying a water-soluble gel or by depressing the air/water valve and allowing the water to run over the distal tip.

Throughout the examination, prevent any excessive bending or twisting of the insertion tube or universal cord. Also be aware of the distance between the control head and the light source so that the light source is not accidentally pulled from its support.

Cleaning, disinfecting and sterilizing

Immediately following an endoscopic examination, the equipment should be thoroughly cleaned to prevent caking of secretions on the soft rubber insertion tube and the interior of the accessory channel. When cleaning these instruments, follow manufacturer's instructions. However, some generalizations can be made.

If the endoscope is fully immersible, as many of the newer models are, the entire control head can be immersed and cleaned as well. If, however, the endoscope is nonimmersible, use a slightly damp cloth to clean the control head. Avoid getting the control head wet. Endoscope seals are not watertight, and fluid can enter and severly damage the fiber system.

The exterior surface of the endoscope can be washed with a mild surgical soap solution (20% soap, 80% water) and a soft cloth or brush. If there is a distal rubber hood present, remove and clean it as well. Rinse the endoscope thoroughly with clean water, then a second time with a 70% alcohol and 30% water mixture.

Clean the interior of the endoscope by immersing the distal tip in the soap solution and suctioning it through the system. Use the cleaning brush provided with the endoscope to dislodge any foreign material adhered to the interior surface of the accessory channel. Clean water can then be suctioned through the system followed by a 70% alcohol/30% water mixture. If a suction pump is not available, flush the solutions through the accessory channel by using the tubing and adapter (that fits the channel opening) provided with the endoscope.

After cleaning and rinsing the endoscope, dry it by suctioning air through the system. Store the endoscope in a hanging position to allow any extra fluid to drain out. The water bottle should be sterilized and stored in a similar way.

Use glutaraldehyde or mild iodophor solutions to disinfect the endoscope. Consult the manufacturer for recommended disinfectants and disinfecting procedures.

A host of cleaning and disinfecting aids are available, ranging from simple trays that function as a third hand during the cleaning process to fully automatic cleaners and disinfectors complete with timers and minicomputers. These are very useful accessories in a practice where numerous endoscopic examinations are performed. Endoscope manufacturers can recommend the cleaning aids best designed for their endoscopes.

The fiberoptic endoscope can also be sterilized if infectious dis-cases are suspected. Ethylene oxide can be used to sterilize the endoscope, but some of the accessories can be placed in the steam autoclave. Follow the manufacturer's instructions on temperature and pressure requirements, aeration times, and presterilization procedures.

PURCHASING THE ENDOSCOPE

When purchasing fiberoptic endoscope equipment for the first time, ask for a demonstration of various models from several manufacturers before making the final decision. Actual use during the demonstration allows one to see the images produced, assess the fit of the instrument in the primary user's hands, determine the ease of operation and observe other desired characteristics necessary for the daily use of the equipment. Discussions with others owning similar equipment can give insight into the advantages and disadvantages of each system. (Table 1-1.)

When the decision is made to purchase equipment from a particular manufacturer, the person who can help the most is the company's area representative. This person can guide a prospective client into purchasing the proper endoscope and light source and all additional accessories the practice will require. Instructions for care, cleaning, maintenance, and future additions to the system also can be obtained from the representative. In addition, this person knows when used equipment (usually from human hospitals and practices)

TABLE 1-1 Some current endoscope model numbers, manufacturers and characteristics

MODEL NUMBER	WORKING LENGTH (MM)	OUTSIDE DIAMETER (MM)	CHANNEL DIAMETER (MM)
Pediatric			
Olympus GIF-P10	1025	9.0	2.0
Olympus GIF-XQ10	1025	9.8	2.8
Pentax FG-29H	1050	9.8	2.8
Pentax FG-23H	1050	7.8	2.1
Fujinon UGI-PE	1110	7.8	2.2
Fujinon UGI-FP3	1110	9.5	2.7
Adult			
Olympus GIF-Q10	1030	11.0	2.8
Pentax FC-34FH	1500	11.5	3.5
Pentax FC-38SH	1150	12.8	3.8
Fujinon UGI-F4	1110	11.0	2.8
Fujinon COL-MP2 (LP2)	1475 (1735)	11.5	3.2

ENDOSCOPE AND ACCESSORY MANUFACTURERS

Major fiberoptic endoscope manufacturers

Olympus Corporation
4 Nevada Drive
Lake Success, NY 11042-1179
516-488-3880

Fujinon Inc.
10 High Point Drive
Wayne, NJ 07470
201-633-5600

Pentax Precision Instrument
Corporation
30 Ramland Rd.
Orangeburg, NY 10962-2699
914-365-0700

Major endoscope accessory manufacturers

Olympus Corporation
4 Nevada Drive
Lake Success, NY 11042-1179
516-488-3880

Fujinon Inc.
10 High Point Drive
Wayne, NJ 07470
201-633-5600

Pentax Precision Instrument
Corporation
30 Ramland Rd.
Orangeburg, NY 10962-2699
914-365-0700

Mill-Rose Laboratories, Inc.
7310 Corporate Boulevard
Mentor, OH 44060-4885
216-255-7995

Hartford Veterinary Supply
Company
9110 Persimmon Tr. Rd.
Potomac, MD 20854
301-299-6031

Video endoscope manufacturers

Welch Allyn Inc.
State Street
Skaneateles Falls, NY
800-445-6567

Olympus Corp.
4 Nevada Drive
Lake Success, NY 11042
516-488-3880

Pentax
30 Ramland Rd.
Orangeburg, NY 10692-2699
800-431-5880

Fujinon Inc.
10 High Point Dr.
Wayne, NJ 07470
800-872-0196

Freeze Frame Recorder
Polaroid Corp.
784 Memorial Drive
Cambridge, MA 02139
800-225-1618

becomes available. This equipment is generally in very good condition and can be purchased at a reasonable price. The current endoscope model numbers, their manufacturers, and some of their characteristics are listed in Table 1-1.★ There are many other models available, but those listed are found to be the most versatile and best suited for equine pediatric and adult endoscopic examinations. Because prices change frequently, they will not be addressed.

★For a list of major endoscope and accessory manufacturers, see box on p. 14.

Chapter 2

VIDEO ENDOSCOPY

MICHAEL J. MURRAY

Video endoscopy is a technology that was applied in human gastroenterology within the past few years[1] and has recently become available for use in veterinary medicine. Its initial veterinary application was in endoscopy of the equine patient, and currently video endoscopy is available in a large number of veterinary clinics, for use in both large and small animals. The technology offers several features that represent advantages over fiberoptic technology, although these features will not be required by all users of endoscopic equipment. This chapter covers the technical aspects of video endoscopy, video endoscopic equipment that is available, and a comparison of the advantages and disadvantages of fiberoptic versus video endoscopic equipment.

PRINCIPLES OF VIDEO ENDOSCOPY

The primary difference between fiberoptic and video endoscopy is in how the image is produced. With conventional fiberoptic endoscopes, the object is illuminated by a standard light source, the image is transmitted through a system of lenses and dedicated glass fibers, and the image is then viewed through an objective lens. With video endoscopy, object illumination, object imaging, and image processing are all coordinated electronically, and the image is viewed on a video monitor.

For video systems used in equine endoscopy, a 300 watt xenon lamp provides the light source. To produce a color image, the light

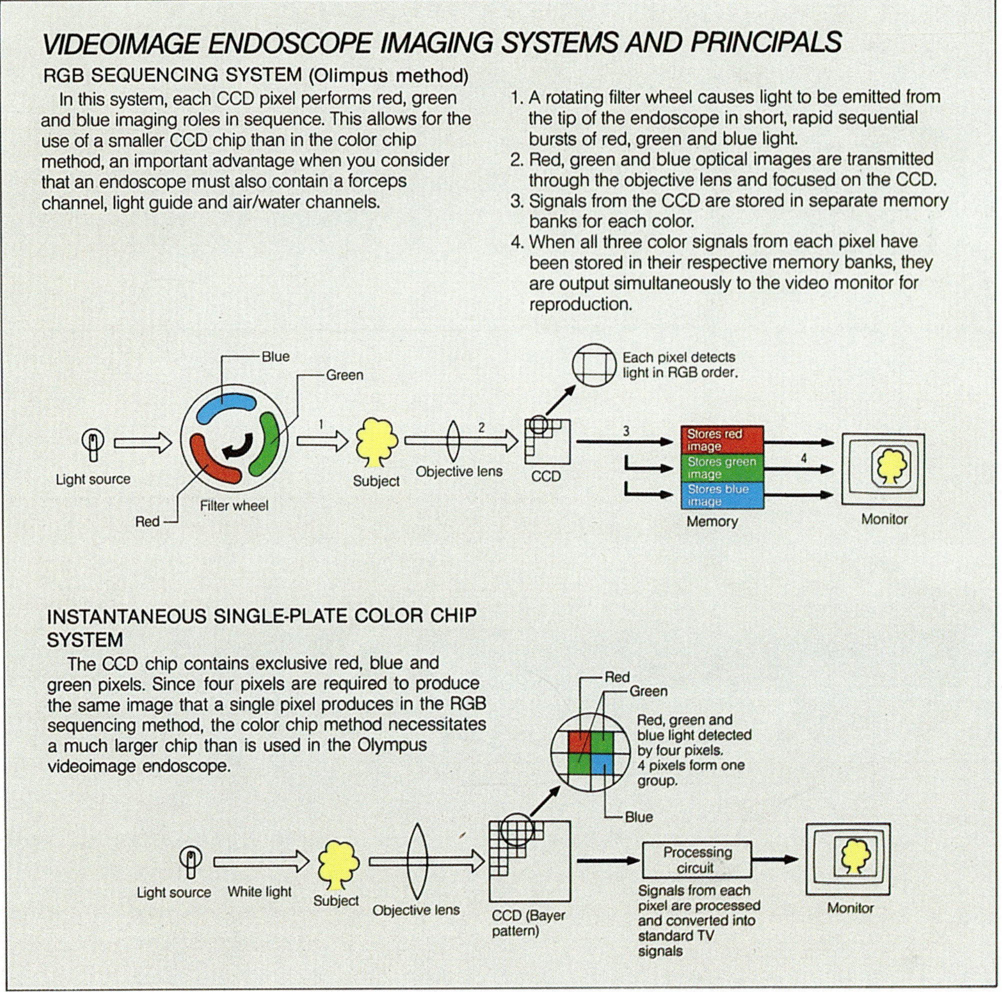

FIG. 2-1 **Principles** of video imaging systems.

(Courtesy Olympus Corporation, Lake Success, New York.)

is passed through a rotating color wheel, with red, green, and blue filters in sequence (Fig. 2-1). The color wheel spins at 20 rotations per second, generating rapid, sequential bursts of red, green, and blue light. This is transmitted down the insertion tube of the endoscope along randomly aligned glass fiber bundles.

The illuminated image is transmitted through an objective lens, which focuses the image onto a charge coupled device (CCD). The CCD is a chip with a grid containing approximately 32,000 pixels. This chip transmits a black and white image. Each pixel "sees" a red, green, or blue image, in sequence, 20 times per second. The amplitudes of red, green, and blue light are different, and thus each sequential impulse illuminating the CCD pixels has a different amplitude corresponding to its color wavelength. The CCD converts this amplitude to an electronic signal that is transmitted back to the video processor, where all of the signals are reassembled into the appropriate color image. The image is displayed on a video monitor and can be recorded on videotape, optical disk, or still image recording equipment.

A color CCD chip, which does not employ a red, green, blue color sequence because the pixels on the chip record the color of the illuminated image directly, produces an image that is superior to that produced by the black-and-white CCD chip. However, the color chip is significantly larger, and thus requires a large endoscope insertion tube diameter (13 to 15 mm) that is unsuitable for many of the applications of endoscopy in equine medicine. Additionally, the color chip technology is currently unavailable in the United States.

The focal length of the endoscope varies with the field of view. With a 90 degree field of view, the focal length is 5 to 100 mm. This depth of field is accomplished by using a small objective lens aperture, identical to the depth of field principle in photography.

VIDEO ENDOSCOPE SYSTEMS

Several manufacturers currently produce video endoscopy equipment (Fig. 2-2), but the equipment available for use in the equine patient is limited at this time. Companies that produce video-endoscopy equipment include Welch Allyn, Olympus, Fuji, Pentax, and Toshiba.★ Welch Allyn is the only American manufacturer of video endoscope systems, and Toshiba is the only manufacturer of an endoscope that utilizes a color chip. However, Toshiba products are prohibited from being sold in the United States at this time. Welch Allyn also is the only manufacturer that produces and markets a video endoscope that is suitable for many of the applications of endoscopy in the horse. Other companies, including Fujinon, Olympus, and Pentax have indicated a willingness to special order endoscopes of sufficient dimensions for use in many of the applications of endoscopy in equine practice.

Welch Allyn manufactures a video endoscope that is 200 cm in working length and 9.5 mm in outer diameter, with a 2.8 mm diameter biopsy channel. This endoscope can be used in endoscopy of the upper and lower airways, the guttural pouches, the male lower urinary system, the female urogenital system, the stomach and duodenum of foals, and the stomach of adult horses. However, a longer endoscope is required for duodenoscopy (310 cm) in the majority of adult horses, and currently a video endoscope of this length is unavailable.

★See box on p. 14 for addresses of these video endoscope manufacturers.

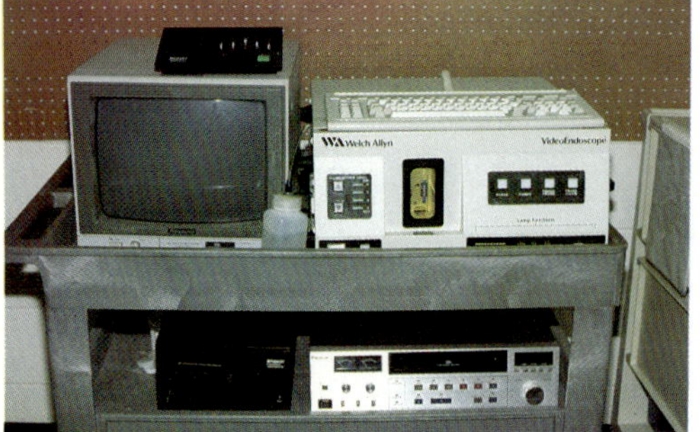

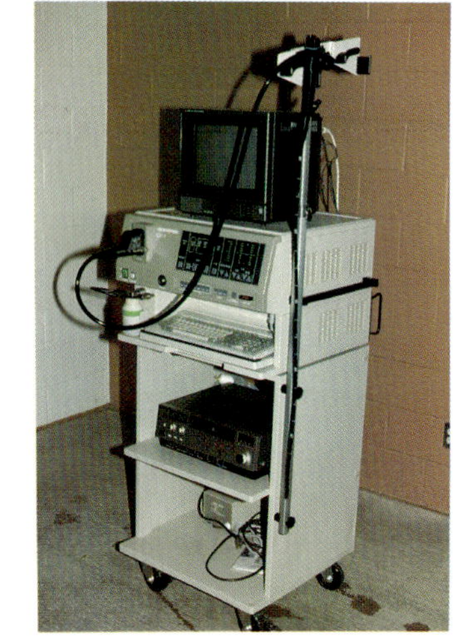

FIG. 2-2 **Two video endoscopy systems.** The Welch Allyn system **(A)** consists of the video processor, keyboard, and color video monitor. Equipment that has been added to the system shown includes a video cassette recorder and a freeze frame recorder, seen on the lower shelf of the cart. The Olympus system **(B)** consists of similar components, although the processor is larger and much heavier than the Welch Allyn processor.

All of the manufacturers produce video endoscopy equipment that is designed for applications in human gastroenterology. These applications include colonoscopy, gastroscopy, and duodenoscopy. Consequently, the equipment that is available includes colonoscopes (65 to 180 cm insertion tube length, 12.5 to 13.8 mm outer diameter, 3.0 to 4.2 mm diameter biopsy channel), gastroscopes (100 to 110 cm length, 9.5 to 11.8 mm outer diameter, 2.8 to 3.7 mm diameter biopsy channel), and duodenoscopes (125 cm length, 10.8 to 12.5 mm outer diameter, 2.8 to 4.2 mm diameter biopsy channel, side-viewing). The colonoscopes are too short to reach the stomach of an adult horse and, generally, too wide to be passed through the ventral nasal meatus of young foals or into the guttural pouch of adults. Colonoscopes would be restricted to use in the upper airway, male lower urinary system, and female urogenital system. The gastroscopes are too short to reach the stomach of foals other than neonates, and would be restricted to use in the upper airway, guttural pouches, male lower urinary system, and female urogenital system. The side-viewing duodenoscopes would have little application in equine endoscopy.

The video endoscope systems include the video processor, a data entry keyboard for display of patient name and pertinent data, and a video monitor. There are some differences in the quality of the image produced by the different systems available,[2,3] although each utilizes the same CCD chip. Also, there are differences in the features and accessories available.

With the Welch Allyn system, for instance, the freeze frame function is controlled from a button on the processor or by a foot pedal. The Olympus and Pentax systems have the freeze frame function controlled via a button on the endoscope control section and also have a button on the endoscope control section to activate the VHS video recorder that they sell as an accessory. The accessories that are available vary between manufacturers, and Olympus has the most complete array of accesories. Accessories that are useful include a cart, a VHS video recorder, still image camera, biopsy instruments, cleaning/disinfecting equipment, suction pump, and air/water peristaltic pump. Other accessories, including ERCP (Endoscopic Retrograde Cholangiopancreatography) cannulae, mechanical lithotriptor, diathermic snares, aspiration biopsy needles, etc. are available from some manufacturers.

In some equine referral practices endoscopic laser surgery is being performed. Welch Allyn produces a laser-compatible endoscope (1.1 meter length, 11.8 mm outer diameter), and the Olympus and Pentax gastroscopes and colonoscopes are laser-compatible. The Welch Allyn and Pentax video processor also can be adapted for use with arthroscopic equipment.

The costs of the systems are relatively similar among manufacturers, with the exception of the more expensive color chip system. The cost of the Welch Allyn system, which includes the Video Processor II, keyboard, Sony monitor, and 200 cm endoscope, is approximately $28,000. The cost of the Olympus system, which includes the video processor, keyboard, cart, endoscope hanger, and Sony monitor, is $13,700 without the endoscope, with an additional $11,200 to $14,700, depending on the endoscope purchased. Although not currently available, a 200 to 300 cm length endoscope would be more expensive. The addition of a video tape recorder and a freeze frame recorder to the system can add $2,500 to $3,500 to the cost of the system.

The Pentax video endoscope system is priced similarly to Olympus and Welch Allyn, but is designed to link up with a computerized data management system. This system stores images in the computer, and these images can be recalled and converted to hard copy at any time. This data management system lists for $14,500.

VIDEO ENDOSCOPY IN USE

With the exception of how one views the endoscopic image, the use of video endoscopic equipment is similar to that of fiberoptic systems. There is no eyepiece with video systems, and the image is displayed on a video monitor. Depending on the type of recording equipment that accompanies the system, one can simultaneously record the examination on video tape, slide or print film, or optical disk. The maneuverability of the endoscope depends on the specific equipment. An endoscope that has a 100 cm insertion tube length will generally have a greater maximum deflection than a 200 cm endoscope, and an endoscope that is 10 mm in outer diameter will have greater flexibility than one with a 12.5 mm outer diameter. Other specifications, such as focal distance and field of view, will vary among manufacturers and specific products within a manufacturer's product line.

Cleaning, disinfecting, and storage of video endoscopes is similar to fiberoptic endoscopes, and specific instructions vary between products and manufacturers. For example, Olympus and Pentax video endoscopes are completely immersible in water, including the control section, while only the insertion tube of the Welch Allyn video endoscope is immersible. Welch Allyn and Olympus video endoscopes can be gas sterilized.

VIDEO VERSUS FIBEROPTIC ENDOSCOPY

Several factors are involved in the consideration of whether to choose a video or fiberoptic endoscopy system (Fig. 2-3). Several of the advantages and disadvantages of each system are listed in Table 2-1, reflecting to some degree the bias of the author. The primary factor is, in fact, the preference of the endoscopist. Comparison of the gastrointestinal endoscopy services of major human medical centers reveals a split in the preference between video and fiberoptic equipment, with several hospitals using solely fiberoptic equipment, and others relying on video endoscopy systems.

The cost of the system will be of major importance. Video systems are 25% to 100% more expensive than fiberoptic systems, depending on the quality of the fiberoptic system. Also of importance is the portability of an endoscope system. Video systems are large and heavy, because of the video processor. The Welch Allyn system is somewhat portable, while the Olympus system is not. Fiberoptic systems vary, but the basic light sources are very portable.

Electronic imaging systems provide a distinctly superior image, compared with most fiberoptic systems, and because the image is not dependent on dedicated glass fibers, image defects from damaged fibers are not a problem. Video systems also have an advan-

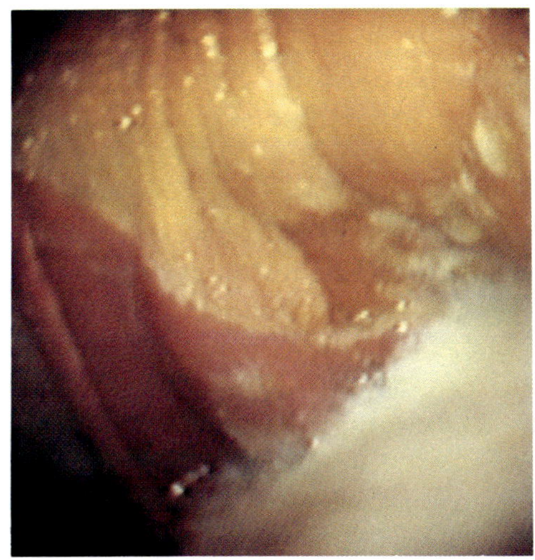
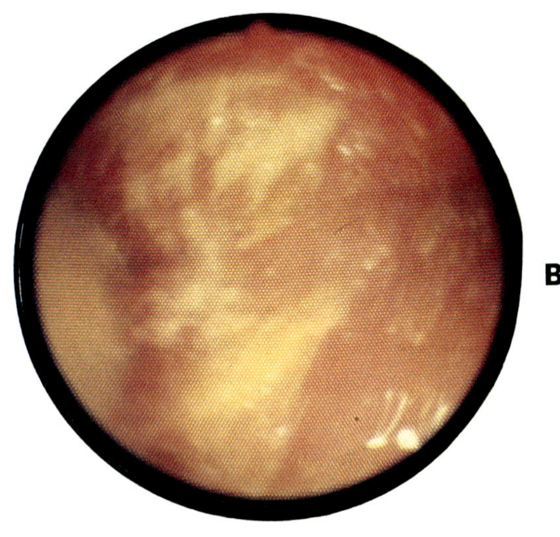

FIG. 2-3 **Comparison of still images** from gastroscopic examinations of horses recorded directly from video endoscope **(A)** and fiberoptic endoscope **(B).** The image from the video endoscope is superior in its clarity, size of the field of view, and capability for recording information pertinent to the examination on the video monitor. This information is included on hard copies of the video image.

TABLE 2-1 A comparison of fiberoptic and video endoscopic systems

FEATURE	PREFERRED SYSTEM
Image quality	Video
Image recording	Video
Still image production	Video
Durability	Video★
Disinfection capabilities	Similar†
Teaching capabilities	Video
Cost	Fiberoptic
Portability	Fiberoptic
Available accessories	Similar

★Overall, video systems are more durable, since minor fiberoptic breakage does not affect image. However, durability will vary with the length and outer diameter of the specific endoscope used.

†Some endoscopes, both video and fiberoptic, are completely immersible in water and disinfecting/sterilizing solutions. Immersibility will be dependent on the manufacturer.

tage in client relations and in teaching. While fiberoptic systems can be modified to produce a video image, modification adds expense to the system, and the image is of poorer quality than with a video system. However, the Pentax fiberoptic endoscope can be connected to a Pentax video processor, which permits the use of either a fiberoptic or video endoscope with this system. This would be of greatest advantage to a practice that already has Pentax fiberoptic endoscopy equipment.

The ability to allow clients to observe the endoscopic examination and to record the examination for further explanation and discussion with the client, colleagues, and/or students is a very important advantage of the video systems. Clients are always very impressed with the quality of the image, and involving the client in the examination enhances the clinician's interaction with the client. Similarly, the video endoscopy system greatly augments instruction for students, interns and residents, and colleagues in veterinary practice.

Another important consideration in acquiring endoscopy equipment is servicing the equipment. Video systems are technically more complex than fiberoptic systems and, thus, could require more frequent and expensive servicing. Replacing an endoscope tip with a video chip costs more than $6000! The type of service contract offered, convenience of service to the customer, and reputation of the manufacturer for providing service should be determined before purchasing endoscopy equipment, fiberoptic or video.

Endoscope durability depends on the length, outer diameter, and use of the equipment. Generally, an endoscope with a smaller outer diameter and a longer length is less durable. Additionally, narrower endoscopes are more flexible and more easily manipulated by a horse's pharynx, such that the horse may flip the endoscope insertion tube into its oral cavity. This is true of both video and fiberoptic endoscopes. Since video endoscopes do not rely on dedicated glass fibers for image transmission, they should be somewhat more durable than comparably sized fiberoptic endoscopes.

The decision of whether to invest in a video endoscopy system will depend on several factors. As more teaching hospitals and private practices acquire video systems, their popularity will likely increase. The bottom line for an individual in private practice will be to determine whether the video system serves both the professional and economic needs of the practice.

REFERENCES

1. Sivak MV: Videoendoscopy, Clin Gastroenterol 15:205, 1986.
2. Knyrim K and others: Optical performance of electronic imaging systems for the colon, Gastroenterology 96:776, 1989.
3. Satava RM: A comparison of direct and indirect video endoscopy, Gastrointest Endosc 33:69, 1987.

Chapter 3

Nasal Cavity

FRANK A. NICKELS

Rhinoscopy is a very important aid in diagnosing diseases of the nasal cavity. Some diseases of the rostral aspect of the nasal cavity can be evaluated by a thorough physical examination (visual and digital), but direct inspection of the more caudal region is possible only with the use of a fiberoptic endoscope. For the purpose of this discussion, only rhinoscopy will be emphasized, as it relates to the diagnosis of diseases of the nasal cavity.

RESTRAINT

The endoscopic examination of the nasal cavity is performed with the animal standing, with minimal physical restraint in most cases. Chemical restraint is rarely indicated except for those horses who are nervous or fractious.

EQUIPMENT

The use of a standard (11 mm) colonoscope is adequate to examine the nasal cavity of mature full-size horses, but in foals and miniature horses, a pediatric bronchoscope or gastroscope (7 to 8 mm) is necessary to examine the entire area.

TECHNIQUE

Developing a routine technique for the examination of the nasal cavity will ensure completeness. If a problem of the nasal cavity is suspected, both sides should be inspected. A useful technique is to examine the ventral meatus, ventral concha, and ventral aspect of the nasal septum as the fiberoptic endoscope is being inserted, and the caudal fundus, the middle meatus, the dorsal concha and the dorsal aspect of the septum as it is being withdrawn.

NORMAL ENDOSCOPIC ANATOMY

The nasal cavity is divided into two similar halves by the median nasal septum and the vomer. The entrance to each nasal cavity is the nostril. The exit from each is the choana. The major portion of each half of the nasal cavity is occupied by the nasal conchae, which project medially from the lateral wall.

The dorsal concha (Fig. 3-1) occupies the dorsal aspect of each nasal cavity. It extends from the cribriform plate of the ethmoid bone to the level of the first cheek tooth. A fold of mucous membrane, the straight fold, extends from the rostral end of the dorsal concha to the nostril. This straight fold (Fig. 3-6) consists of two rounded ridges, of which the dorsal contains the cartilaginous extension of the concha.

The ventral concha (Figs. 3-1, 3-2, 3-4, and 3-5) is shorter than the dorsal. It extends from the level of the sixth cheek tooth to the level of the first cheek tooth. A fold of mucous membrane extends from the rostral end of the ventral concha on the lateral wall of the nasal cavity to the prominence formed in the medial wing of the nostril by the lamina of the alar cartilage. Another fold, the ventral or basal fold, extends rostroventrally from the rostral end of the ventral nasal concha and parallels the nasal process of the incisive bone. The dorsal and ventral concha divide the outer part of the nasal cavity into three meatuses: dorsal, middle, and ventral.

The dorsal meatus (Figs. 3-4 and 3-5) is a narrow passage bound dorsally by the roof of the nasal cavity and ventrally by the dorsal concha. The middle meatus (Figs. 3-1, 3-2 and 3-4) lies between the dorsal concha and the ventral concha and is somewhat smaller than the dorsal meatus. The communication between the nasal cavity and maxillary sinus (nasomaxillary opening) is in the caudal part of this meatus. The nasomaxillary opening is a narrow, slit-like opening that is not visible from the nasal side. The ventral meatus (Fig. 3-5) is bound dorsally by the ventral concha and the ventral floor of the nasal cavity. It is a larger passage than either the dorsal or middle meatus and leads directly into the nasopharynx.

The common meatus (Fig. 3-6) is the space between the nasal septum and the conchae and between the roof and the floor of the nasal cavity. The space is widest on the floor of the nasal cavity.

Endoturbinate II (Figs. 3-1 to 3-3) and the ethmoid nasal conchae (endoturbinate III and IV) (Fig. 3-3) are the visible structures of the ethmoid labyrinth that project rostral into the caudal part of the nasal cavity. Between the ethmoturbinates are three principal passages and numerous small passages—the ethmoidal meatuses. Endoturbinate I (Figs. 3-1 and 3-3) is dorsal to the other endoturbinates and is the largest. Endoscopically, endoturbinate I appears to be the caudal extent of the dorsal nasal concha.

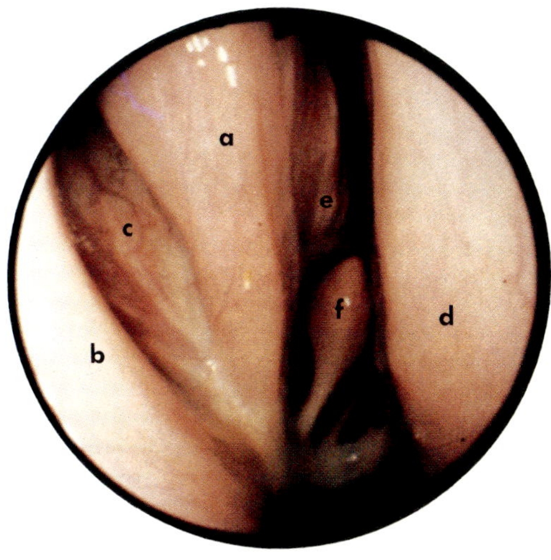

FIG. 3-1 Dorsocaudal area of the nasal cavity. Dorsal concha *(a)*; ventral concha *(b)*; middle meatus *(c)*; nasal septum *(d)*; Endoturbinate I *(e)*; Endoturbinate II *(f)*.

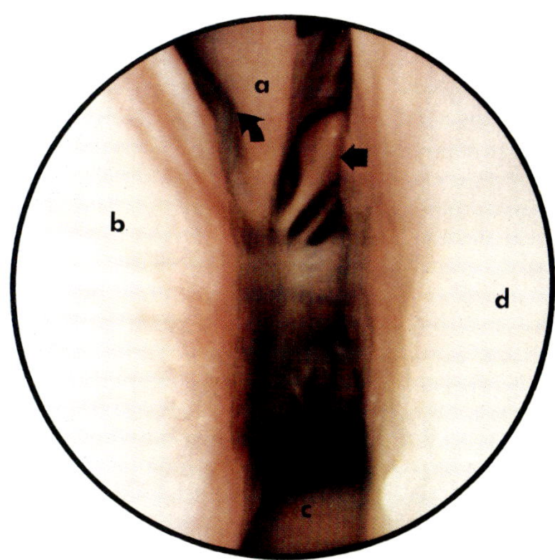

FIG. 3-2 Ventrocaudal area of the nasal cavity. Dorsal concha *(a)*; ventral concha *(b)*; middle meatus (curved arrow); Endoturbinate II *(straight arrow)*; soft palate *(c)*; nasal septum *(d)*.

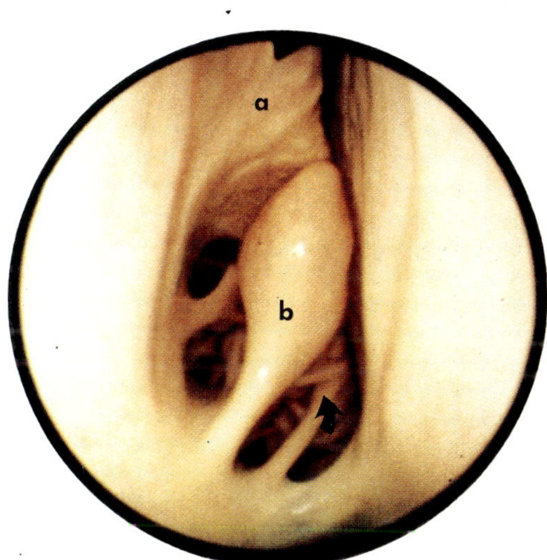

FIG. 3-3 Endoturbinates. Endoturbinate I *(a)*; Endoturbinate II (b); Endoturbinate III to V *(curved arrow)*.

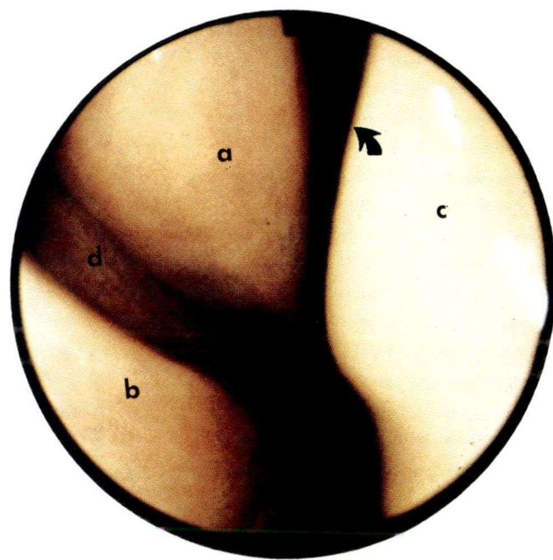

FIG. 3-4 Dorsal middle area of the nasal cavity. Dorsal concha *(a)*; ventral concha *(b)*; nasal septum *(c)*; dorsal meatus *(curved arrow)*; middle meatus *(d)*.

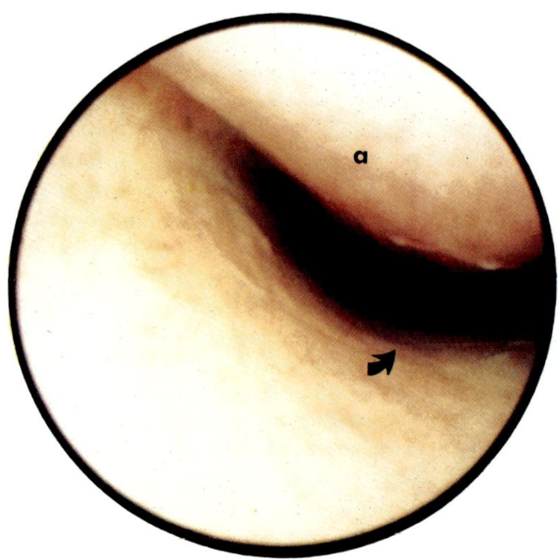

FIG. 3-5 Ventral concha *(a);* ventral meatus *(curved arrow).*

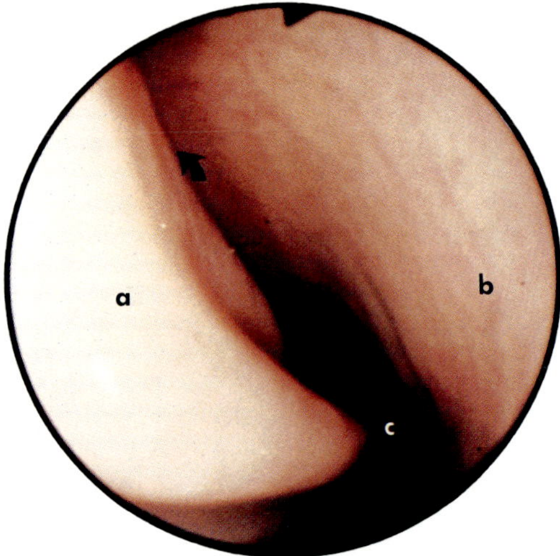

FIG. 3-6 Dorsorostral area of the nasal cavity. Dorsal meatus *(curved arrow);* straight fold of dorsal concha *(a);* nasal septum *(b);* common meatus *(c).*

DISEASES OF THE NASAL CAVITY

Diseases of the external nares and nasal cavity (Table 3-1) are important because these structures provide the only normal passage for airflow to and from the respiratory tract in the horse. Other species change to mouth breathing during exercise to decrease upper airway resistance, but the horse is unique because it maintains nasal breathing during exercise and is unable to do otherwise. Although the upper airway accounts for only a small fraction of the total airway resistance in the normal horse, diseases of the external nares and nasal cavity increase airway resistance. Fortunately, diseases of this portion of the upper airway are not frequent.

Diseases of the nasal cavity are usually characterized by a unilateral or bilateral obstruction that reduces airflow and may cause a nasal stertor. These obstructions can be caused by diseases of the mucosal surfaces, nasal conchae, or nasal septum or expanding lesions within the paranasal sinuses. The other most common clinical sign is a unilateral nasal discharge. This discharge can range from a

TABLE 3-1 Diseases of the nasal cavity which may be diagnosed endoscopically

CONDITION	CLINICAL SIGNS
Nasal polyps	Usually unilateral; cause reduced airflow and occasional nasal discharge.
Ethmoid hematoma	Intermittent epistaxis or serosanguineous nasal discharge; large ones cause obstruction (Fig. 3-7)
Granuloma	May be fungal in origin (e.g. cryptococcus); nasal discharge and obstruction (Fig. 3-10)
Foreign bodies	Often sudden onset; hemorrhage and nasal discharge
Skull fractures	May involve nasal passages, hemorrhage and nasal obstruction (Fig. 3-12)
Fistula	Rare, following trauma or tooth loss (Fig. 3-13).
Sinusitis	Various causes; exudate discharges into middle meatus (Fig. 3-9)

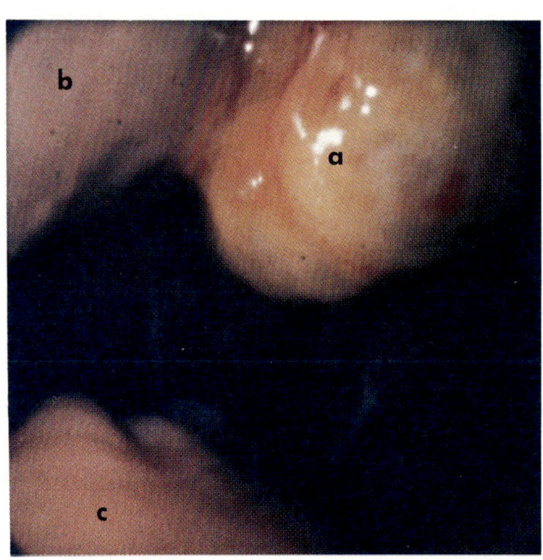

FIG. 3-7   Ethmoid hematoma *(a)*; nasal septum *(b)*; soft palate *(c)*.
(Courtesy Dr RP Hackett, Cornell University.)

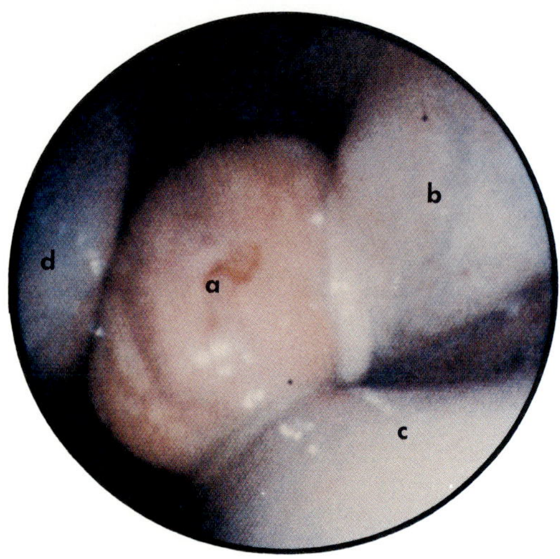

FIG. 3-8   Myxosarcoma *(a)*; dorsal concha *(b)*; ventral concha *(c)*; nasal septum *(d)*.
(Courtesy Dr RP Hackett, Cornell University.)

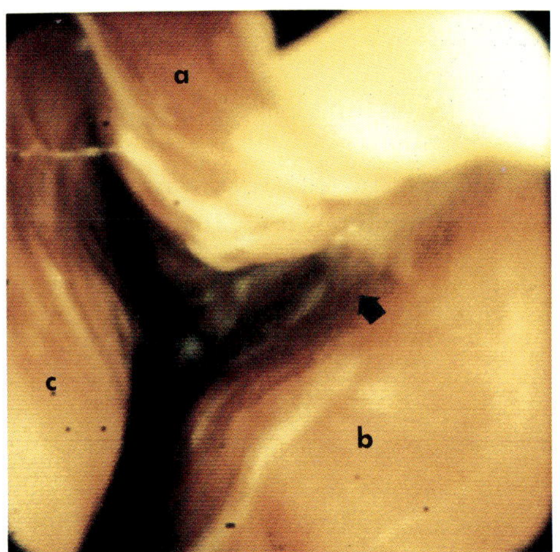

FIG. 3-9   Exudate draining from nasomaxillary opening *(straight arrow)*; exudate on the dorsal concha *(a)*; ventral concha *(b)*; and nasal septum *(c)*.
(Courtesy Dr RP Hackett, Cornell University.)

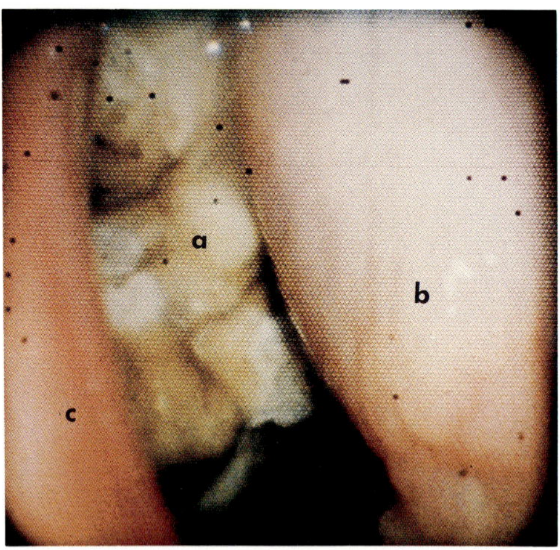

FIG. 3-10   Fungal granuloma *(a)*; nasal septum *(b)*; ventral concha *(c)*.

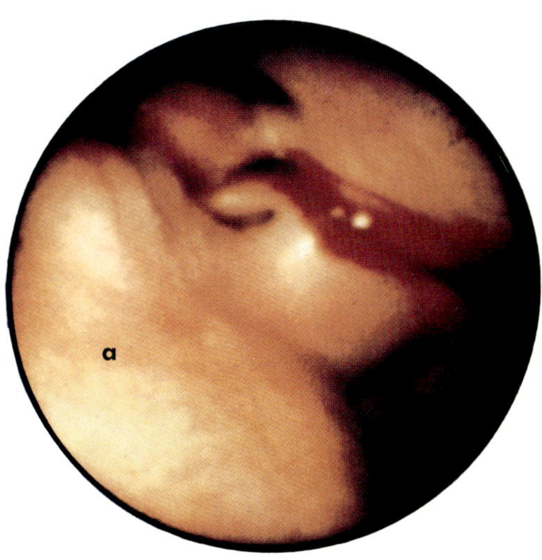

FIG. 3-11   Hemorrhage from ethmoidal meatus. Nasal septum *(a)*.

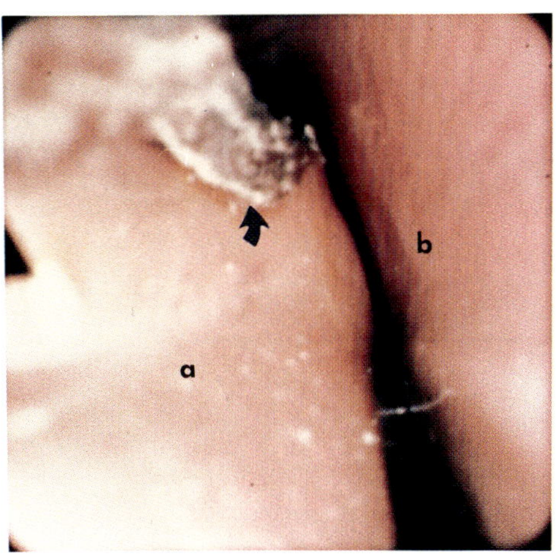

FIG. 3-12   Penetration of fracture segment of the nasal bone into dorsal meatus *(curved arrow)*; dorsal concha *(a)*; nasal septum *(b)*.

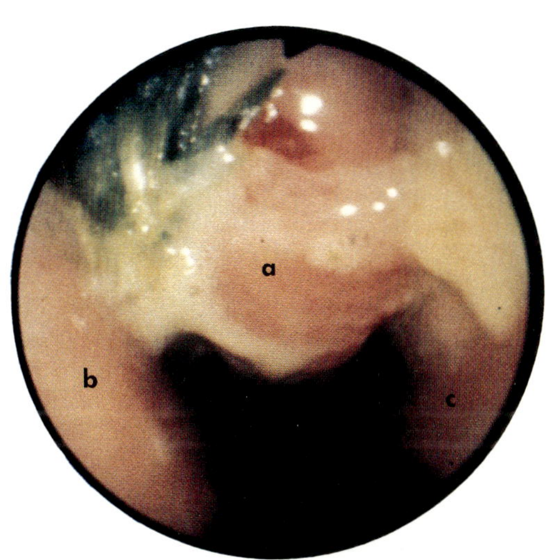

FIG. 3-13   A rim of granulation around a nasomaxillary fistula *(a)*. Feed material is adhered to the surface. Nasal septum *(b)*; ventral concha *(c)*.

serous discharge to a mucopurulent or serosanguineous discharge. Occasionally, facial distortion or a fetid odor may be present if the condition is in advanced stages.

Most conditions of the external nares and rostral nasal cavity can be diagnosed by a thorough physical examination, whereas others require a more detailed examination with radiography and endoscopy.

Chapter 4

PHARYNX

JOSEPH J. BERTONE

RESTRAINT AND TECHNIQUES

Restraint considerations are paramount to the examination of the pharyngeal area of horses. The restraint methods used for pharyngeal examination depend on the disposition of the horse, the duration of the examination, and the specific portion of the pharynx to be evaluated. A complete pharyngeal examination requires that the endoscope be passed through a naris for nasopharyngeal and dorsal laryngopharyngeal examinations and through the mouth for oropharyngeal and ventral laryngopharyngeal examinations (see Figs. 4-1 to 4-4 for anatomy).

The nasopharynx and dorsal laryngopharynx (Figs. 4-1 to 4-3) are examined by advancing the endoscope through either nostril and through the associated nasal cavity to a length of 30 to 40 cm. Physical restraint techniques (e.g., halter restraint, firm grasp of the bridge of the nose, lip twitch, skin twitch, and ear hold) are often sufficient to examine these cavities in tolerant horses. The initial insertion of the endoscope is often the portion of the examination horses contend with most. Care should be exercised, since some horses strongly object to this procedure. The tolerance of horses to endoscopic examination of the upper airways can be evaluated by inserting a finger into the naris and observing the incited reaction. Less tolerant horses may require some form of chemical restraint (e.g., acetylpromazine maleate, xylazine hydrochloride) to decrease

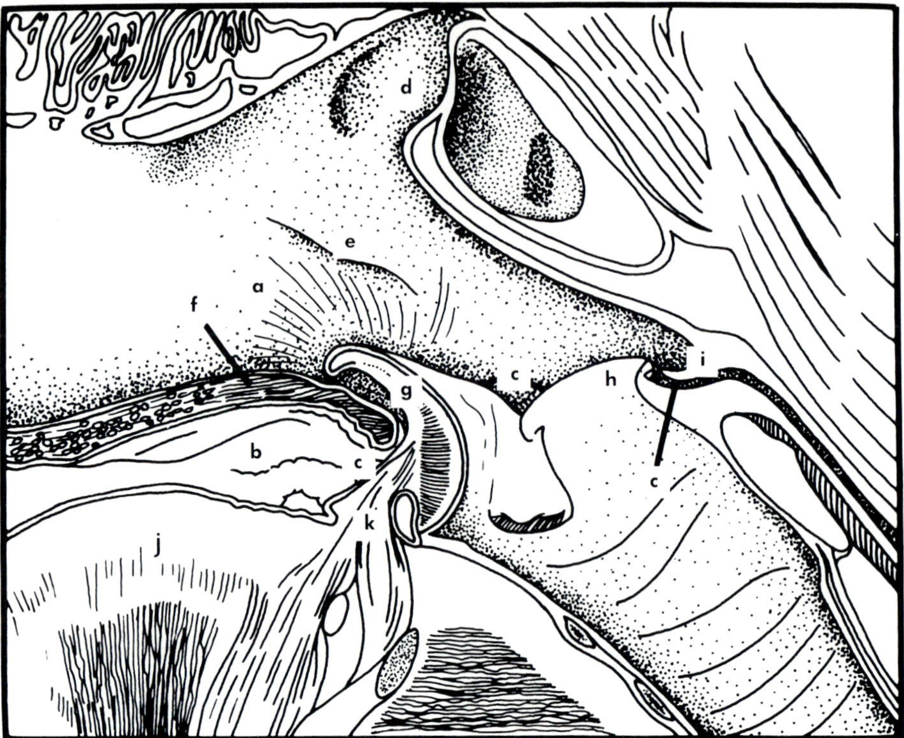

FIG. 4-1 Sagittal section of the pharynx of the horse. *a,* Nasopharynx; *b,* oropharynx; *c,* laryngopharynx; *d,* dorsal pharyngeal recess; *e,* pharyngeal opening of the auditory tube; *f,* soft palate; *g,* epiglottis; *h,* corniculate process of the arytenoid cartilage; *i,* palatopharyngeal arch; *j,* base of the tongue; *k,* glossoepiglottic fold.

the risk of operator injury and equipment damage. The operator should look through and guide the endoscope while advancing it to decrease the risk of trauma to the nasal mucosa or the nasal and ethmoid conchae. Maximal restraint is needed for examination of the oropharynx and ventral laryngopharynx, since the endoscope must be advanced through the mouth and oral cavity. It is recommended that this procedure be performed in conjunction with general anesthesia. Use of an oral speculum, gag, or other aid to keep the mouth open will decrease the risk of harm to equipment and operator. A tubular speculum or endotracheal tube may be used to pass the endoscope through the narrow passageway between the dental arcades.

ANATOMY

The three portions of the pharynx include the nasopharynx, oropharynx, and the laryngopharynx (Figs. 4-1 to 4-4).[11,15] The

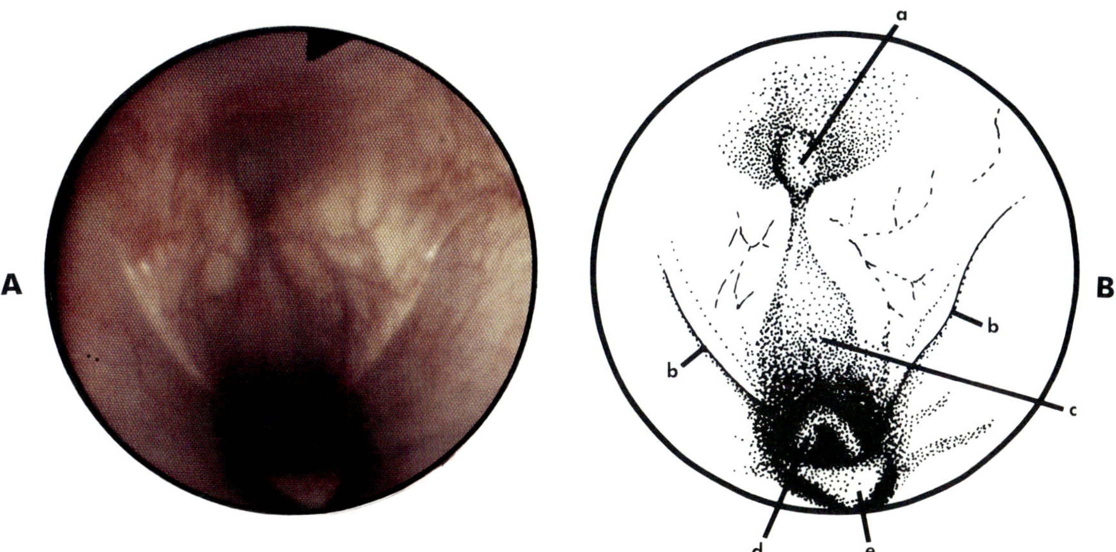

FIG. 4-2 **Nasopharynx. A,** Endoscopic view of the nasopharynx from the rostral extent of the nasopharynx. **B,** Illustration of endoscopic view of the nasopharynx as in **A.** *a,* Dorsal pharyngeal recess; *b,* pharyngeal openings of the auditory tubes; *c,* tubal tonsil; *d,* corniculate process of the arytenoid cartilage; *e,* epiglottis.

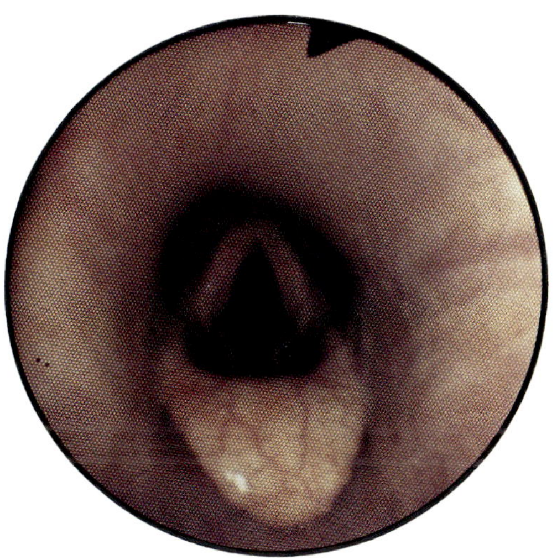

FIG. 4-3   **Dorsal laryngopharynx.** Endoscopic view from the nasopharynx. The dorsal laryngopharynx is dorsal to the intrapharyngeal opening and extends to the level of the cricoid cartilages and contains the rostral structures of the larynx.

soft palate divides the rostral pharynx in a dorsal plane. The **nasopharynx** (Fig. 4-1 and 4-2) is part of the respiratory tract and is dorsal to the soft palate, extending from the choanae to the rostral border of the intrapharyngeal opening. The pharyngeal openings of the auditory tubes (guttural pouch openings) are located on the lat-

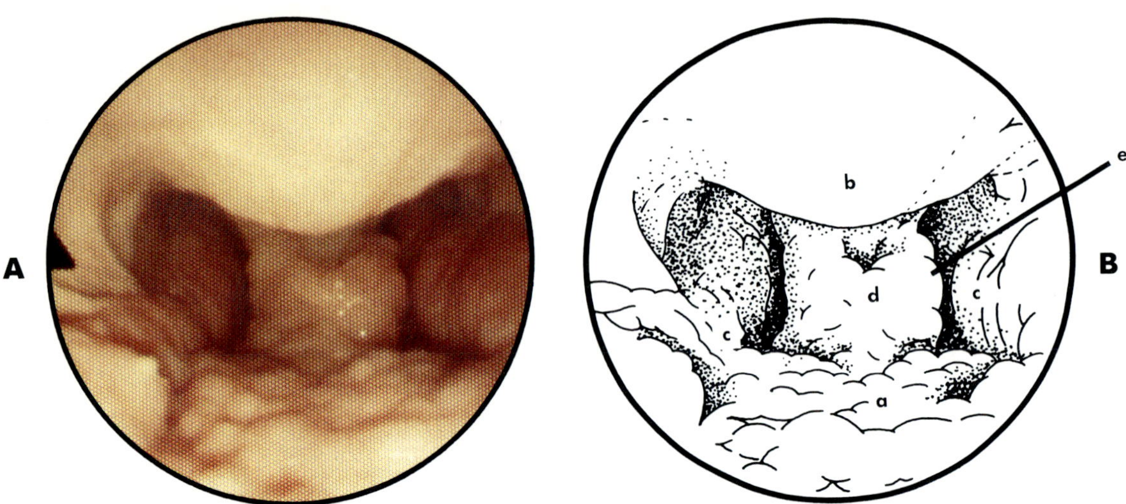

FIG. 4-4 Oropharynx and ventral laryngopharynx. A, Endoscopic view from the oral cavity of the oropharynx and ventral laryngopharynx when the epiglottis is in its normal position. **B,** Illustration of endoscopic view from the oral cavity of the oropharynx and ventral laryngopharynx when the epiglottis is in its normal position as in **A,** *a,* Lingual tonsil blanketing root of the tongue; *b,* soft palate; *c,* palatoglossal arch; *d,* glossoepiglottic fold; *e,* piriform recess. **C,** Endoscopic view from the oral cavity of the oropharynx and ventral laryngopharynx when the epiglottis has been displaced ventrally by endotracheal intubation. **D,** Illustration of the endoscopic view from the oral cavity of the oropharynx and ventral laryngopharynx when the epiglottis is displaced ventrally as in **C.** *a,* Root of the tongue with lingual tonsil; *b,* soft palate; *c,* palatoglossal arch; *d,* glossoepiglottic fold; *e,* piriform recess; *f,* epiglottis; *g,* palatine tonsil.

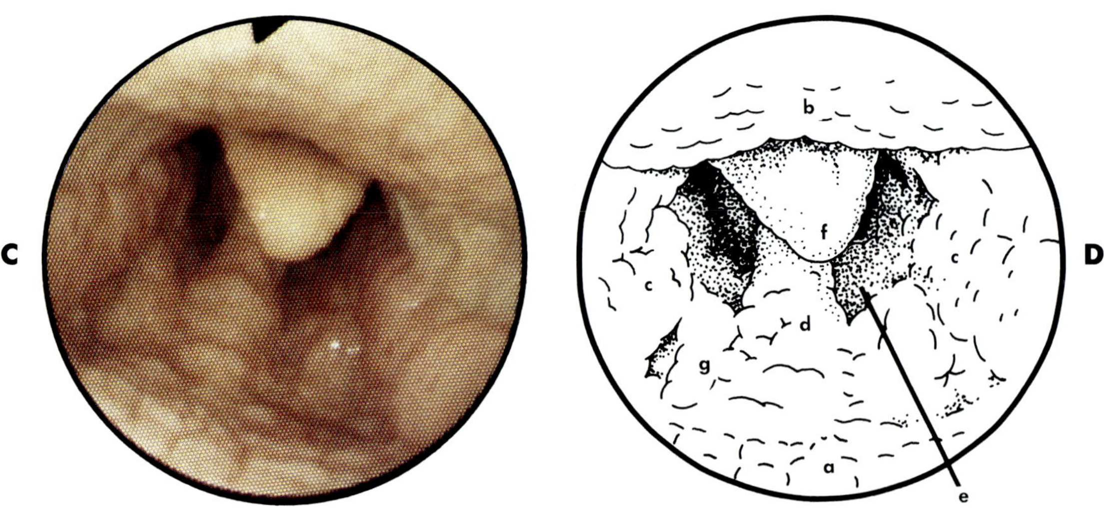

eral walls of the nasopharynx. Although these openings are commonly termed the guttural pouch openings, the guttural pouches (diverticula tubae auditivae) open into the auditory tubes, and there is no direct connection of the pouches with the pharynx.

The dorsal and ventral boundaries of the **oropharynx** (Figs. 4-1 and 4-4) are the soft palate and the surface of the root of the tongue, respectively. The oropharynx extends rostrally from the pharyngeal entrance at the level of the palatoglossal arches and caudally to the base of the epiglottis. In horses, the oropharynx is almost exclusively part of the digestive tract. Only in specific palatal disorders or under special circumstances (such as coughing) does the oropharynx act as a conduit for air movement between the respiratory tract and the external environment.

The **laryngopharynx** (Figs. 4-1, 4-3 and 4-4) is the crossroad of the digestive and respiratory tracts. It is caudal and adjacent to both the oropharynx and nasopharynx, extending from the base of the epiglottis to the level of the cricoid cartilages. The laryngopharynx contains the rostral structures of the larynx.[11,15]

The pharyngeal structures are covered by mucous membrane, which is corrugated in areas where there are pharyngeal glands and/ or accumulations of lymphatic tissue. Tonsillar tissue (aggregated lymphatic tissue) is located diffusely throughout the pharyngeal mucosa. The aggregated oropharyngeal lymphatic tissue is follicular and includes the lingual and palatine tonsils, and the tonsil of the soft palate. The lingual tonsil (Fig. 4-4) is located at the base of the tongue and spreads across the glossoepiglottic fold. The palatine tonsil (Fig. 4-4) is on the caudoventral surface of the oropharynx, lateral to the glossoepiglottic fold. The palatine tonsil extends rostrally from the base of the epiglottis for 10 to 12 cm. The tonsil of the soft palate is oval and located on the rostroventral surface of the soft palate in the oropharynx. The aggregated nasopharyngeal lymphatic tissue is composed of both diffuse and follicular types and includes the pharyngeal and tubal tonsil. The pharyngeal tonsil is located in the area of the choanae and at the caudal end of the nasal septum. The tubal tonsil (Fig. 4-2, *B*) is found dorsally from the pharyngeal openings of the auditory tubes to ventrally the dorsal surface of the soft palate and continues caudally along the lateral walls of the pharynx into the laryngopharynx.[11,15]

FUNCTIONAL ANALYSIS

The major function of the pharynx is to provide selective movement of air into the trachea and ingesta into the esophagus. Endoscopic examination can aid in the analysis of pharyngeal function by use of the following techniques.

Endoscopic visual examination

Feed particles found in the nasopharynx should increase suspicion of a structural and/or functional defect associated with pharyngeal malfunction.

Induced swallow reflex

With the endoscope in the nasopharynx, the swallow reflex is elicited by spraying a small amount of water through the flushing channel of the endoscope or by advancing the endoscope tip into the vicinity of the dorsal laryngopharynx. If the horse is cooperative, it can be fed hay or grain to elicit the reflex. When the swallow reflex is elicited, a rostrodorsal movement of the soft palate occurs, with a constriction of the nasopharynx. These responses are followed by opening and medial placement of the pharyngeal openings of the auditory tubes. The medial reposition of the pharyngeal openings of the auditory tubes is sufficient for their medial aspects to come very close to or even touch each other. Movement of the soft palate and action of the pharyngeal openings of the auditory tubes are probably associated with the actions of the levator and the tensor veli palatini and stylopharyngeus muscles. When the nasopharynx is viewed from the nasal passage during swallowing, the rostrodorsal placement of the soft palate obscures the view of the caudal nasopharynx, larynx, and dorsal laryngopharynx (Fig. 4-5). When the reflex is completed, no feed particles should be seen in

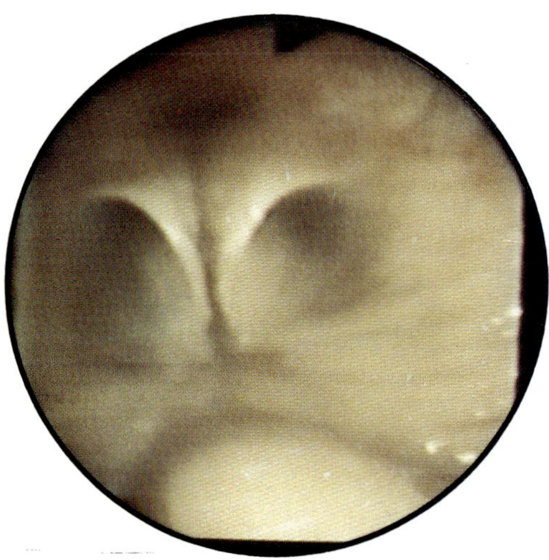

FIG. 4-5 Swallow response. Endoscopic view from the left rostral nasopharynx. The view of the larynx has been obscured by dorsal placement of the soft palate and constriction of the caudal nasopharynx. The pharyngeal openings of the auditory tubes are open and their free margins placed medially. This photograph was taken from a video endoscope projection. Compare this with Fig. 4-2, A.

the nasopharynx. There is some concern that tranquilizing inhibits the swallow reflex.[9] However, there is no experimental work to support this assumption. If the swallow reflex is to be evaluated endoscopically, tranquilizers should not be used. However, mild sedation may have little or no effect.

TABLE 4-1 Pharyngeal diseases and their associated clinical signs

CONDITION	CLINICAL SIGNS
Pharyngeal lymphoid hyperplasia[1,8,9,13] (Fig. 4-6)	Possible exercise intolerance; upper respiratory noise, particularly in severe cases and with severe exercise; nasal discharge; incidental finding
Dorsal displacement of the soft palate[1,7-9] (Fig. 4-7)	Exercise intolerance and upper respiratory noise with severe exercise, particularly in later stages of work; coughing; nasal discharge; can normally be displaced for a short period after deglutition
Pharyngeal cysts[8-10] (Fig. 4-8)	Possible upper respiratory noise and exercise intolerance; coughing; nasal discharge
Rostral displacement of the palatopharyngeal arch[1,6,8] (Fig. 4-9)	Exercise intolerance; upper respiratory noise; dysphagia; nasal discharge; coughing; weight loss
Pharyngeal paralysis[12]	Dysphagia; nasal discharge often containing food; weight loss
Cleft soft palate[1,8,12] (Fig. 4-10), Hypoplastic soft palate[2] (Fig. 4-11)	Dysphagia; nasal discharge often containing food; coughing, weight loss
Pharyngeal mycosis[3,5] (Fig. 4-12 and 4-13)	Nasal discharge, sometimes hemorrhagic; exercise intolerance; upper respiratory noise; dysphagia; coughing; weight loss
Nasopharyngeal cicatrices[14] (Fig. 4-14)	Exercise intolerance and abnormal phonation, depending upon the severity and position of the lesion
Pharyngeal-guttural pouch fistula (Fig. 4-15)	Nasal discharge; incidental finding
Foreign body, trauma, neoplasia, abscess[1,4,8,12]	Any of the above clinical signs, depending on the location and extent of the lesion

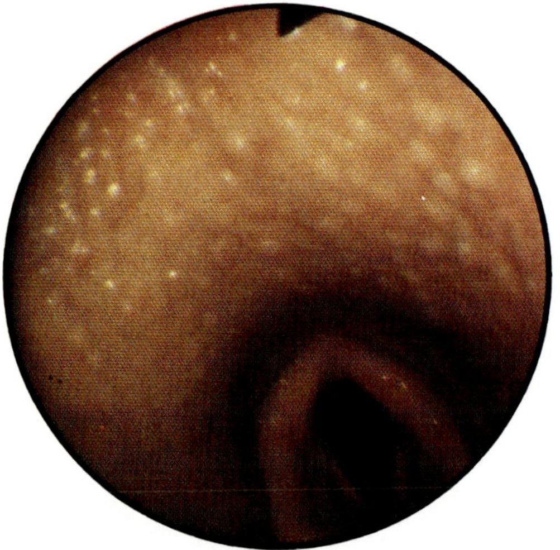

FIG. 4-6 Pharyngeal lymphoid hyperplasia. Endoscopic view from the nasopharynx. There are multiple 2 to 4 mm diameter raised elevations of the surface of the caudal nasopharynx. These lesions would be indicative of Grade 2 lymphoid hyperplasia of the tubal tonsil. Compare this with Fig. 4-3.

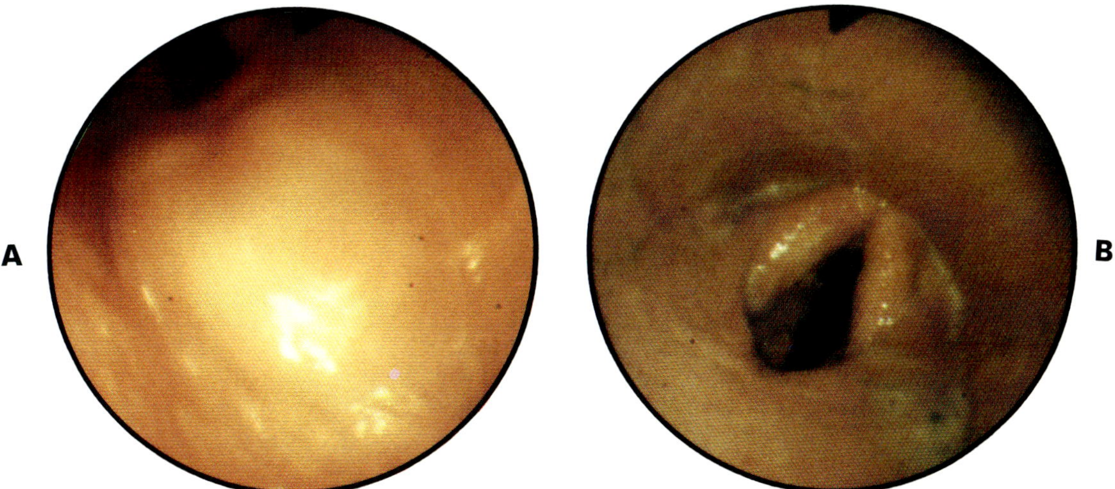

FIG. 4-7 **Dorsal displacement of the soft palate. A,** Endoscopic view from the rostral nasopharynx. The view of the epiglottis is obscured by the soft palate. In this case the displaced epiglottis causes the soft palate to bulge dorsally. **B,** Endoscopic view from the caudal nasopharynx. The view of the epiglottis is obscured by the soft palate. Compare this with Fig. 4-3.

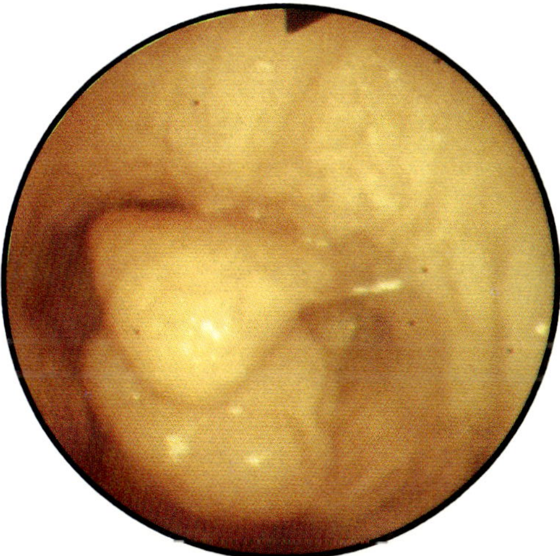

FIG. 4-8 **Pharyngeal cysts.**
Endoscopic view from the nasopharynx. The body and tip of the epiglottis are displaced dorsally because of cystic structures present at the free border of the soft palate. Compare this with Fig. 4-3.

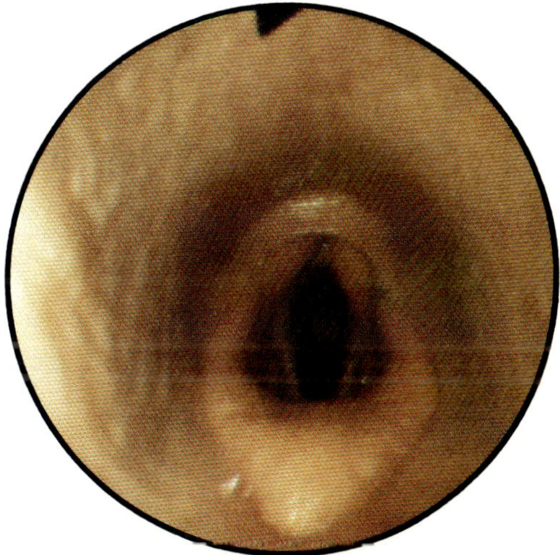

FIG. 4-9 **Rostral displacement of the palatopharyngeal arch.** Endoscopic view from the nasopharynx. The dorsal aspects of the arytenoid cartilages are obscured by the displaced palatopharyngeal arch. Compare this with Fig. 4-3.

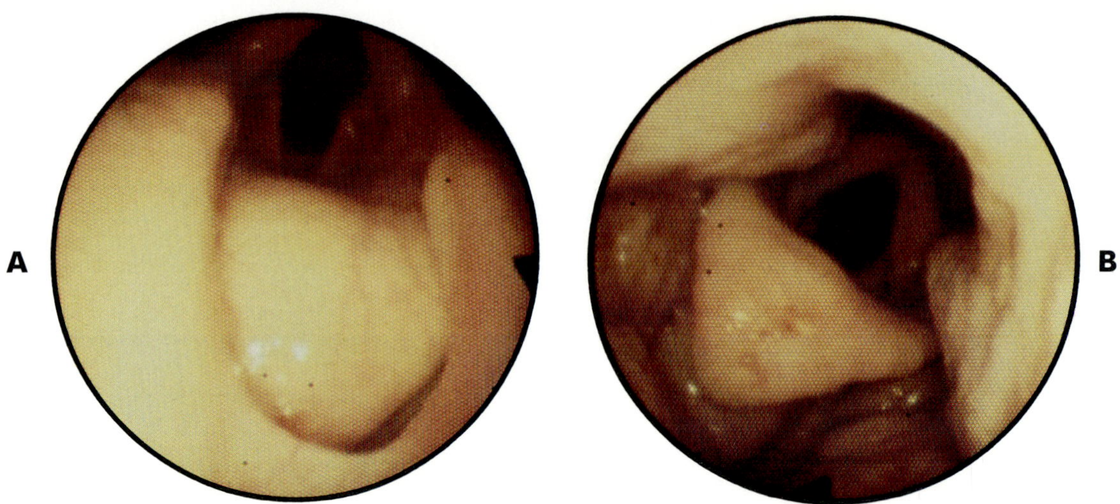

FIG. 4-10 Cleft soft palate. A, Endoscopic view from the nasopharynx. The body of the epiglottis lies in the oropharynx since it is not supported by the soft palate. The epiglottis and borders of the palatal defect are evident. Compare this with Fig. 4-3. **B,** Endoscopic view from the oropharynx. The body of the epiglottis lies in the oropharynx since it is not supported by the soft palate. Compare this with Fig. 4-4.

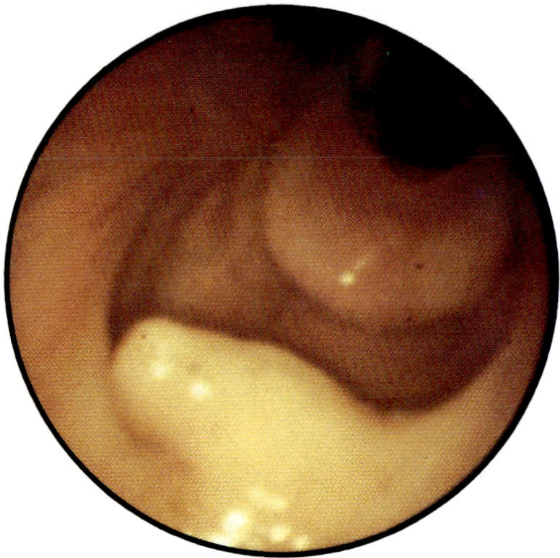

FIG. 4-11 Hypoplastic soft palate. Endoscopic view from the nasopharynx. As with cleft soft palate, the epiglottis is in the oropharynx because of lack of support by the soft palate. The elongated soft palatal structure is analogous to the uvula in human beings. The epiglottis in this case is entrapped by the aryepiglottic fold. Compare this with Fig. 4-3.

(From Bertone JJ et al: J Am Vet Med Assoc 188(7):727, 1986.)

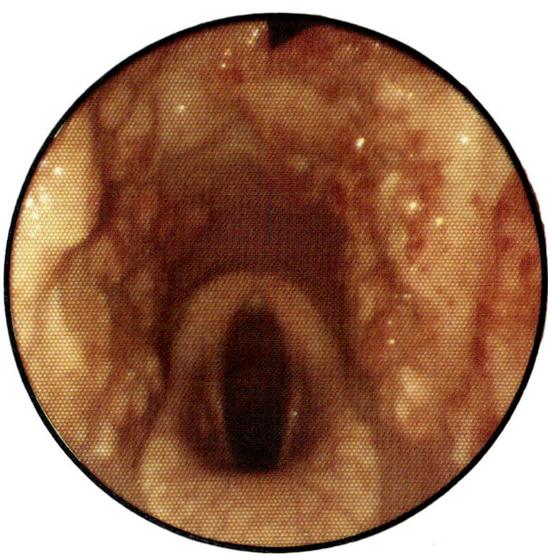

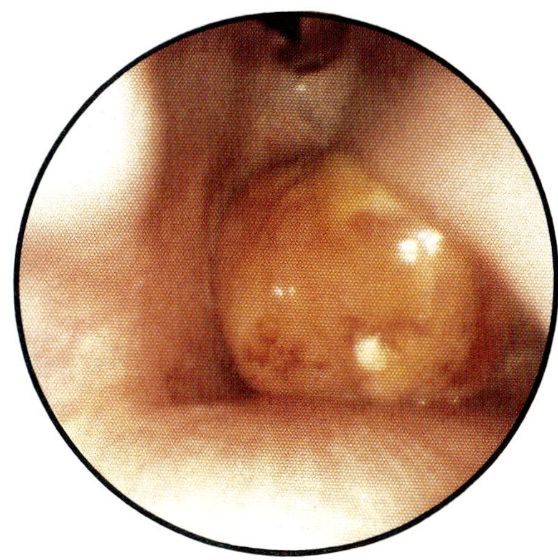

FIG. 4-12   Pharyngeal mycosis.
Endoscopic view from the nasopharynx.
The caudal nasopharyngeal mucosa is
roughened and hemorrhagic rather than
smooth. Often yellow granules are
present on the mucosa. Compare this
with Fig. 4-3.

FIG. 4-13   Cryptococcal rhinitis.
Endoscopic view from the nasal passage.
This mass lies just caudal to the
choanae.

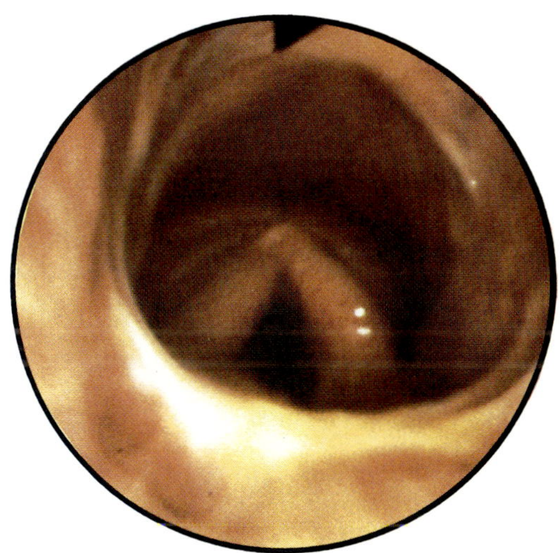

FIG. 4-14   Nasopharyngeal cicatrices.
Endoscopic view from the nasopharynx.
Bands of fibrous tissue are associated
with varying degrees of nasopharyngeal
stenosis. These structures vary in size,
location, and, therefore degree of airway
obstruction. The arytenoid cartilages are
partially obscured by a band of fibrous
tissue along the dorsal surface of the soft
palate. Compare this with Fig. 4-3.
(From Schumacher J and Hanselka DV: J Am
Vet Med Assoc 191(2):239, 1987.)

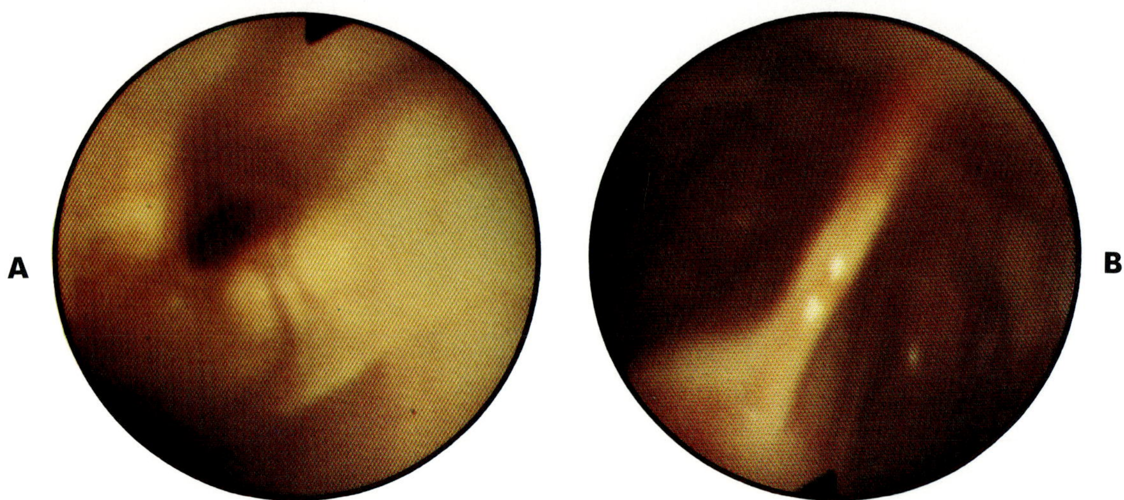

FIG. 4-15 Pharyngeal-guttural pouch fistula. A, Endoscopic view from the nasopharynx. The fistula establishes communication between the dorsal pharyngeal recess and both guttural pouches. The pharyngeal opening of the left auditory tube is evident. Compare this with Fig. 4-2. **B,** Endoscopic view through the fistula. The medial septum between the guttural pouches is evident.

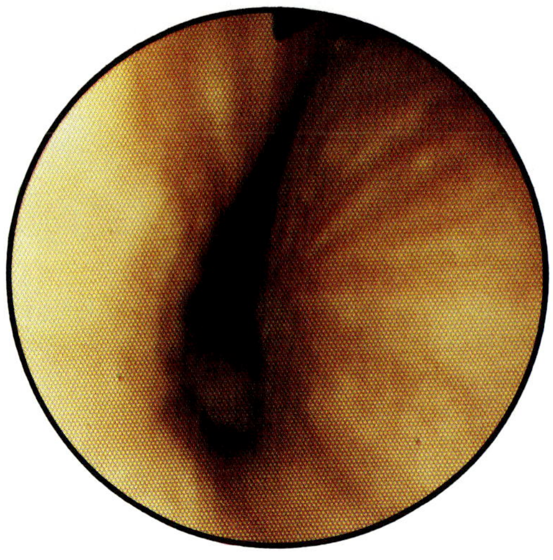

FIG. 4-16 Retropharyngeal airway obstruction. A melanoma in the left guttural pouch has constricted the caudal nasopharynx. Similar obstructions can be associated with other tumors or with abscesses. The tip of the epiglottis can be seen. Compare this with Fig. 4-3.

REFERENCES

1. Baker GJ: Diseases of the pharynx. In Robinson NE, editor: Current therapy in equine medicine, Philadelphia: 1987 WB Saunders Co.
2. Bertone JJ, Traub-Dargatz JL, and Trotter GW: Bilateral hypoplasia of the soft palate and aryepiglottic entrapment in a horse, J Am Vet Med Assoc 188(7):727, 1986.
3. Corrier DE, Wilson SR and Scrutchfield WL: Equine cryptococcal rhinitis, Comp Cont Ed Pract Vet 6:S556, 1984.
4. Dorn CR and Priester WA: Epidemiological analysis of oral and pharyngeal cancer in dogs, cats, horses, and cattle, J Am Vet Med Assoc 169(11):1202, 1976.
5. French DD, Haynes PF, and Miller RI: Surgical and medical management of rhinophycomycosis (conidiobolomycosis) in a horse, J Am Vet Med Assoc 186:1105, 1985.
6. Goulden BE and others: Rostral displacement of the palatopharyngeal arch: a case report, Eq Vet J 8(3):95, 1976.
7. Haynes PF: Dorsal displacement of the soft palate and epiglottic entrapment: diagnosis, management and interrelationship, Comp Cont Ed Pract Vet 5:S379, 1983.
8. Haynes PF: Surgery of the equine respiratory tract. In: Jenning PB, editor: The practice of large animal surgery, Philadelphia 1984, WB Saunders.
9. Koch C: Diseases of the larynx and pharynx of the horse, Comp Cont Ed Pract Vet 2(5):S73, 1980.
10. Koch DB and Tate LP: Pharyngeal cysts in horses, J Am Vet Med Assoc 173:860, 1978.
11. Nickel R and others: The viscera of the domestic mammals, ed 2 Berlin 1973 Verlag Paul Parey.
12. Raker CW: The nasopharynx. In, Mansmann RA, McAllister ES, and Pratt PW, editors: Equine medicine and surgery, Santa Barbara Calif, 1982, American Veterinary Publications, Inc.
13. Raker CW and Boles CL: Pharyngeal lymphoid hyperplasia in the horse. J Eq Med Surg 2:202, 1978.
14. Schumacher J and Hanselka DV: Nasopharyngeal cicatrices in horses: 47 cases (1972-1985), J Am Vet Med Assoc 191(2):239, 1987.
15. Sisson S: Equine digestive system. In Sisson S, Grossman JD and Getty R, editors: The anatomy of the domestic species, Philadelphia 1975, WB Saunders.

Chapter 5

GUTTURAL POUCH

JOHN P. CARON

The guttural pouches are paired auditory (eustachian) tube diverticulae unique to the horse. Located caudally to the pharynx, dorsally to the larynx, and ventrally to the first and second cervical vertebrae, the guttural pouches are related to several cranial nerves, the retropharyngeal lymph nodes, and branches of the common carotid artery and their accompanying veins. Inflammation of or physical damage to the structures adjacent to the guttural pouches accounts for many of the clinical signs observed in guttural pouch disease. Endoscopy is a useful adjunct to physical and radiographic examination and has greatly simplified the diagnosis and treatment of diseases of the guttural pouch.

TECHNIQUE FOR EXAMINATION

Evaluation of the nasopharyngeal opening of the guttural pouch provides limited information regarding the status of its interior. However, more useful information is obtained from direct inspection of the pouch lumen. The volume of the guttural pouch, approximately 300 ml, permits easy endoscopic examination, but the relatively narrow nasopharyngeal opening and proximal auditory tube have to be negotiated before entering the pouch. Thus, a small endoscope (e.g., human bronchoscope (6 mm O.D.)) is often used for guttural pouch examination. Frequently, a conventionally sized instrument (human colonoscope, 11 mm O.D.), may be passed into the guttural pouch. If possible, the use of a larger endoscope is preferred because a larger diameter instrument provides more light and a larger field of view than a smaller endoscope. An endoscope with a biopsy channel and lens rinsing capability is advantageous but not essential.

Endoscopic examination of the gutteral pouches is usually conducted on the standing, sedated horse. To minimize the potential for injury to the horse, handlers, or equipment, the horse is usually restrained in a set of stocks. A lip twitch may be applied.

The endoscope is introduced to the nasopharynx via the ventral nasal meatus. The paired nasopharyngeal openings of the gutteral pouches are inspected for abnormalities of shape or for the presence of discharges (Fig. 5-1). A clear, mucous discharge of modest volume (produced by the respiratory epithelium lining the gutteral pouches) is normal.

Access to the interior of the gutteral pouch is through the nasopharyngeal opening, located on the lateral wall of the nasopharynx, rostral and ventral to the pharyngeal recess. Each opening is slit-like, approximately 3 cm long and concealed by a cartilaginous flap with a caudal base (Fig. 5-1). Introduction of an endoscope into the lumen of the gutteral pouch requires that a second instrument be used to adduct this flap and prevent the tip of the endoscope from being deflected wide of the opening.

Instrument deflection may be prevented by a number of methods. One technique involves the use of a flexible endoscopic biopsy tool. With the tip of the endoscope approximately 2 to 3 cm rostral to the nasopharyngeal opening, the biopsy tool is advanced through the appropriate channel of the endoscope, beneath the flap, and into the gutteral pouch (Fig. 5-2). The biopsy instrument is used as a "guide wire" over which the endoscope is advanced into the pouch lumen. Entry into the pouch is facilitated by rotating the endoscope on its long axis during advancement under the flap. This uses the eccentric location of the biopsy channel to advantage. Rotation of the endoscope adducts the cartilaginous flap and prevents deflection of the endoscope tip into the nasopharynx or its catching on the mucosa of the rostral eustachian tube. The operator views the progress of the endoscope while rotating it back and forth until it enters the pouch lumen. Once inside the pouch, the biopsy instrument is withdrawn.

A second popular technique used to enter the gutteral pouch involves adduction of the flap with a rigid bent-tipped catheter. An equine female urinary catheter (Chambers catheter) is suitable, or a similar device may be fashioned from a disposable insemination pipette. The bent tip of the catheter is advanced through the ventral nasal meatus of the side being examined. The catheter is passed under the cartilaginous flap and rotated to adduct it (Fig. 5-3 and 5-4). The endoscope is directed under or over the catheter shaft, through

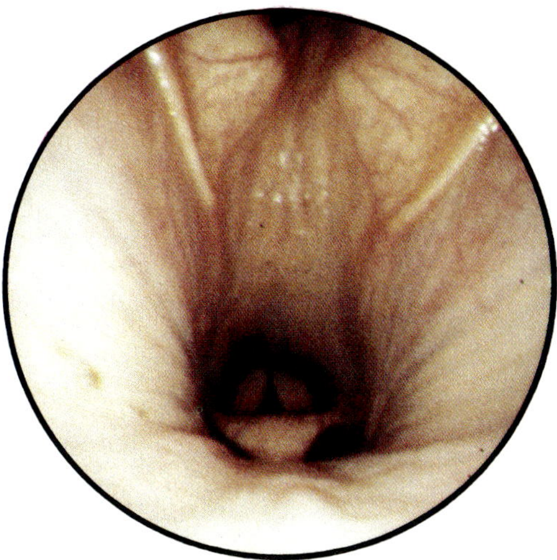

FIG. 5-1 Equine nasopharynx showing the paired nasopharyngeal openings to the guttural pouches, the dorsal pharyngeal recess, and the rostral portion of the larynx. Endoscope tip is at the level of the rostral nasopharynx.

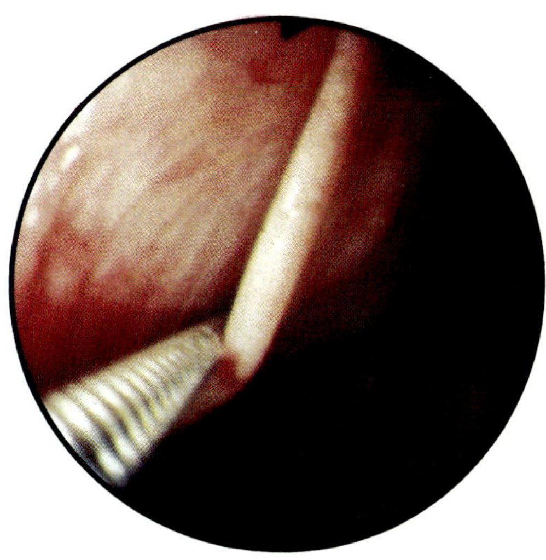

FIG. 5-2 Medial cartilaginous flap of the nasopharyngeal opening of the right guttural pouch with a flexible biopsy instrument introduced into guttural pouch lumen. Endoscope tip is approximately 3 cm rostral to the aperture.

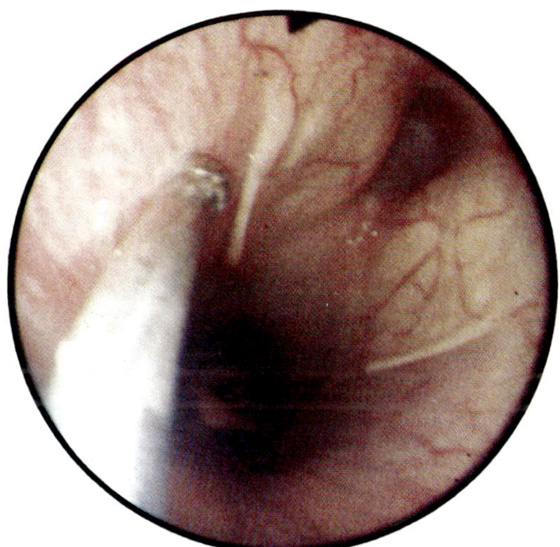

FIG. 5-3 Nasopharynx with Chambers catheter located immediately rostral to nasopharyngeal opening of the right guttural pouch. Catheter is advanced under the flap and rotated to adduct it. Endoscope tip is approximately 6 cm rostral to the aperture.

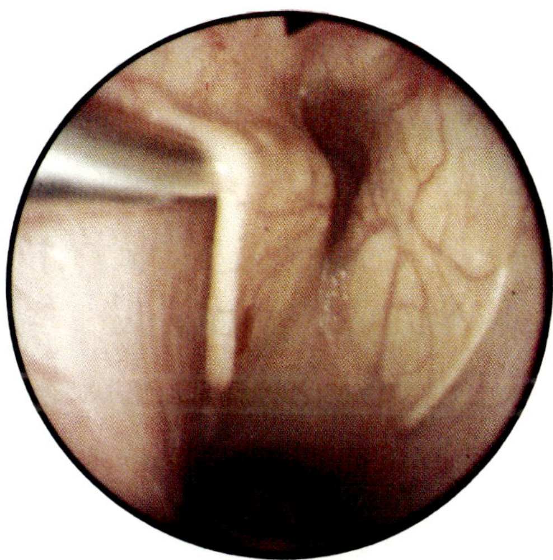

FIG. 5-4 Medial cartilaginous flap of the nasopharyngeal opening of the right guttural pouch partially adducted with a Chambers catheter.

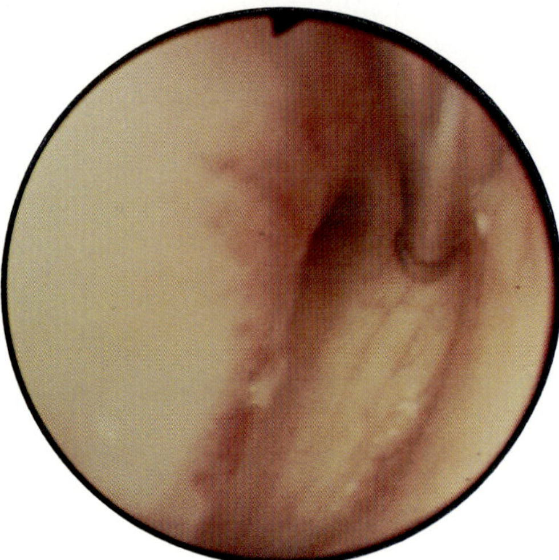

FIG. 5-5   Field of view with the endoscope within the rostral portion of the auditory tube. A Chambers catheter is in contact with the surface of the cartilaginous flap (medial lamina) of the auditory tube.

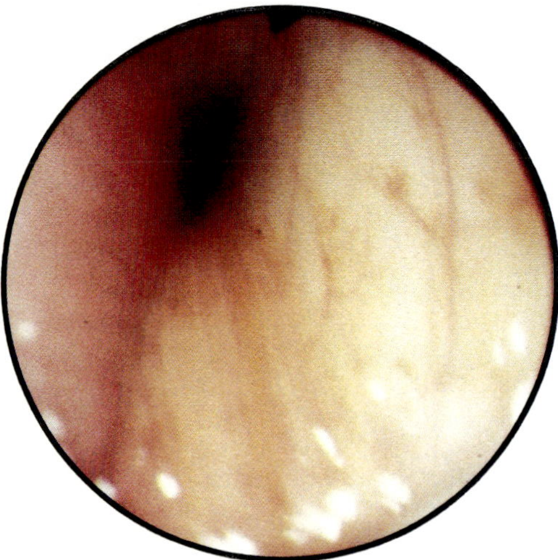

FIG. 5-6   Caudal portion of the rostral auditory tube seen during introduction of the endoscope into the lumen of the right guttural pouch. Endoscope has been advanced beyond the level of the nasopharyngeal flap.

the rostral auditory tube, and into the pouch lumen (Fig. 5-5 and 5-6). The procedure is simplified if the catheter tip is located at either the dorsal or the ventral extremity of the flap to maximize the space available for the endoscope. The catheter is removed once entry into the guttural pouch is confirmed.

During introduction of the endoscope through the rostral auditory tube, the field of view is occupied largely by mucosal folds lining the tube (Fig. 5-6). With either method of introduction, it is helpful to observe the progress of the endoscope while it is being advanced and aim at the dark portion of the field of view (Fig. 5-6). Slowly advancing the endoscope while making small adjustments in the position of its tip, rather than vigorously attempting to introduce the instrument, is more likely to be successful.

In addition, the endoscope can be used to direct the placement of irrigation catheters for the treatment of gutteral pouch empyema.

ENDOSCOPIC ANATOMY

Each guttural pouch consists of two compartments incompletely divided in the sagittal plane by the stylohyoid bone (great cornu) (Fig. 5-7 to 5-12). The stylohyoid bone courses dorsocaudally, invaginating the mucosa of the pouch, and inserts on the styloid process of the petrous temporal bone. It is easily identified by its orientation, its white color, and the presence of the occipitohyoideus muscle attached to its ventromedial surface. The stylohyoid bone is an important anatomic landmark for orientation within the guttural pouch; the mucous membrane of the dorsocaudal medial compartment, adjacent to the stylohyoid bone insertion, is a very frequent site of origin of guttural pouch mycosis.

Inspection of the lateral compartment reveals the external carotid and maxillary arteries (Figs. 5-8 and 5-9). The arteries appear as a single, large, white structure coursing craniodorsally through the lateral compartment. (The arteries are the same vessel; the external carotid artery is known as the maxillary artery, distal to the origin of the superficial temporal artery). A portion of the external maxillary vein is also visible through the mucosa, rostral to the external carotid/maxillary artery (Fig. 5-8).

The volume of the medial compartment is roughly twice that of the lateral compartment and extends further caudally and ventrally. It is also more easily examined than the lateral compartment. Several important structures are located adjacent to the medial compartment. The internal carotid artery and cranial nerves IX, X, XI, XII, the sympathetic trunk, and the cranial cervical ganglion are contained in a fold of the caudolateral wall mucosa of the medial compartment (Figs. 5-10 and 5-11). The fold courses ventrolaterally from adjacent to the stylohyoid insertion and roughly bisects the

Text continued on p. 57

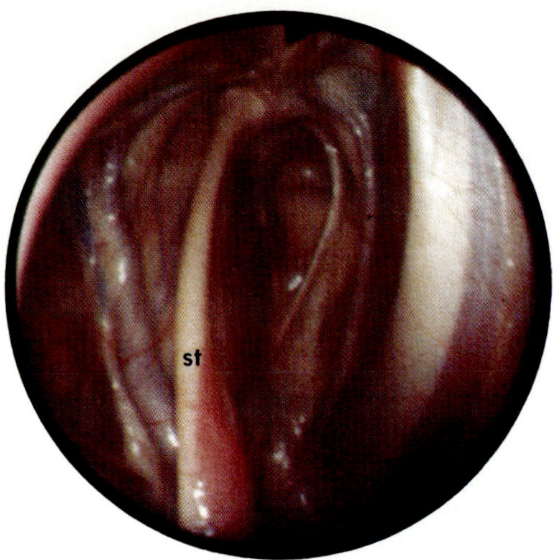
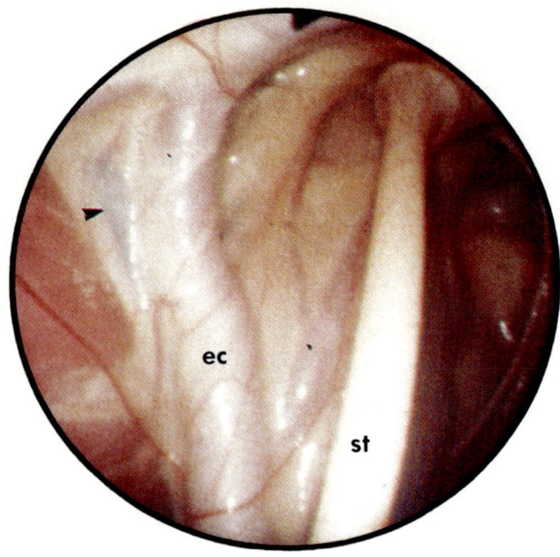

FIG. 5-7 Right guttural pouch viewed from the dorsal and rostral aspect. Endoscope is located immediately caudal to the lumenal entrance of the auditory tube. The stylohyoid bone *(st)* divides the pouch into lateral (left) and medial (right) portions, the stylohyoid-petrous temporal articulation, and is visible caudodorsally.

FIG. 5-8 Dorsal portion of the lateral compartment of the right guttural pouch. The stylohyoid bone is present on the right *(st)* and the external carotid/maxillary artery is visible *(ec),* as is a small portion of the maxillary vein, immediately rostral to the artery *(arrow).*

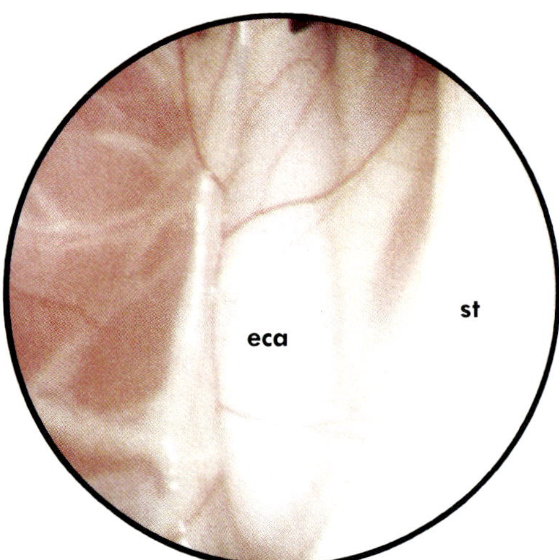

FIG. 5-9 Floor of the lateral compartment of the right guttural pouch. The stylohyoid bone *(st)* and the external carotid *(eca)* are visible.

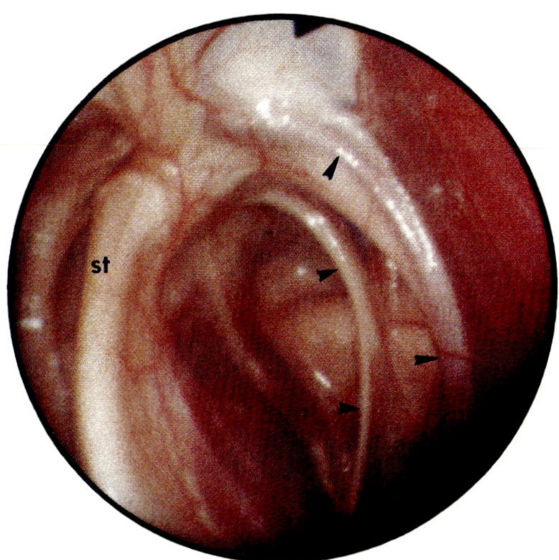

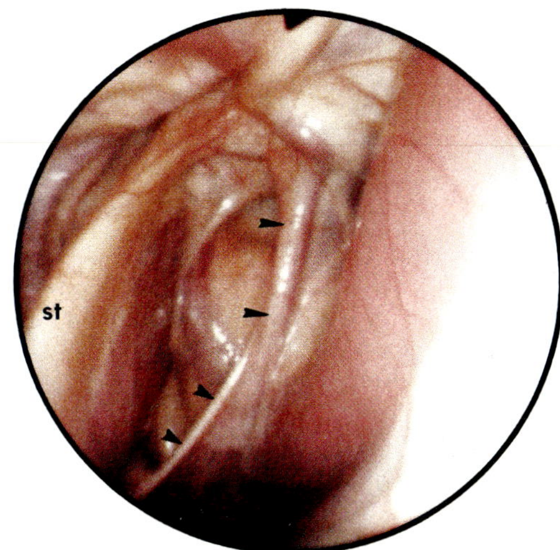

FIG. 5-10 **Dorsocaudal aspect of the medial compartment** of the right guttural pouch. The internal carotid artery *(large arrows [right])* and several cranial nerves coursing dorsoventrally are visible as is the stylohyoid bone *(st).* Small arrows *(left)* indicate cranial nerves IX and XII.

FIG. 5-11 **Dorsocaudal aspect** of the medial compartment of the right guttural pouch. Endoscopic view is similar to Fig. 5-10 but is from a different horse. Notice the more parallel course followed by the internal carotid artery and cranial nerves. Internal carotid artery *(large arrows);* cranial nerves IX and XII *(small arrows);* stylohyoid bone (st).

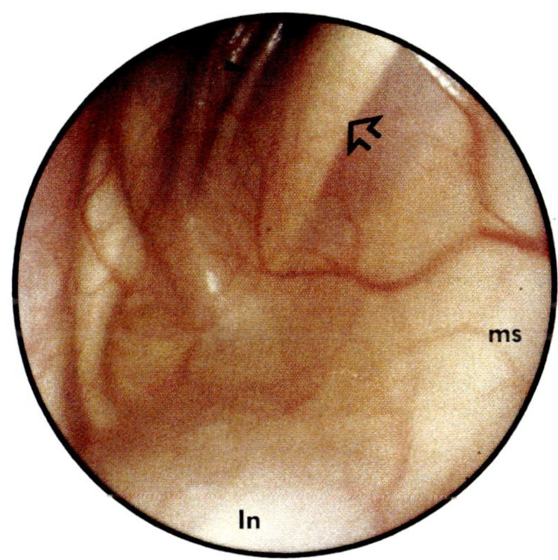

FIG. 5-12 **Floor of the medial compartment.** Internal carotid artery *(small arrow),* tendon of insertion of longus capitis muscle *(open arrow),* and an indentation in the mucosa by a medial retropharyngeal lymph node *(ln)* is evident. The medial septum *(ms)* separates the right and left guttural pouches.

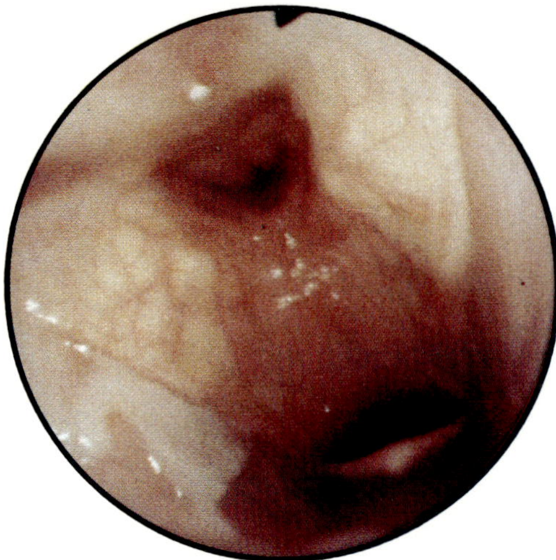

FIG. 5-13 Endoscopic view of nasopharynx in horse with empyema of the right guttural pouch. Note the drainage of exudate from the nasopharyngeal opening.

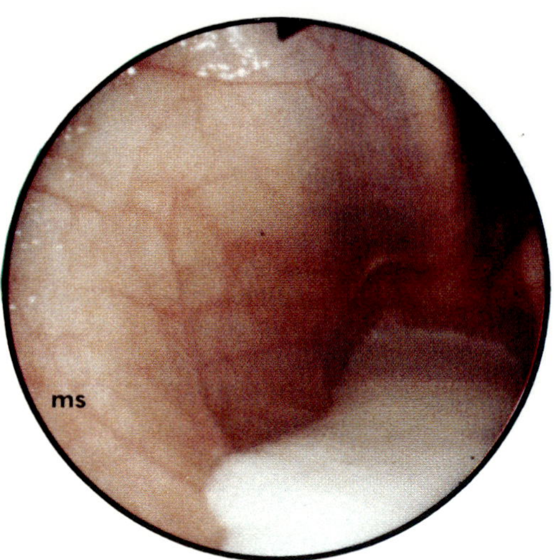

FIG. 5-14 Suppurative fluid on the floor of the medial compartment of a horse with left guttural pouch empyema (*ms* indicates medial septum).

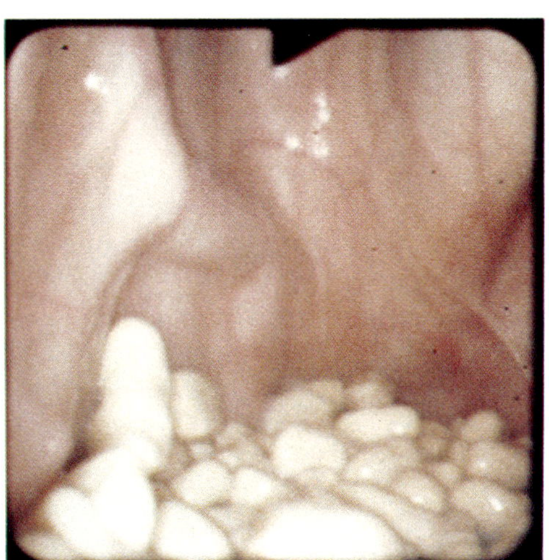

FIG. 5-15 Chondroids in the medial compartment of the left guttural pouch.

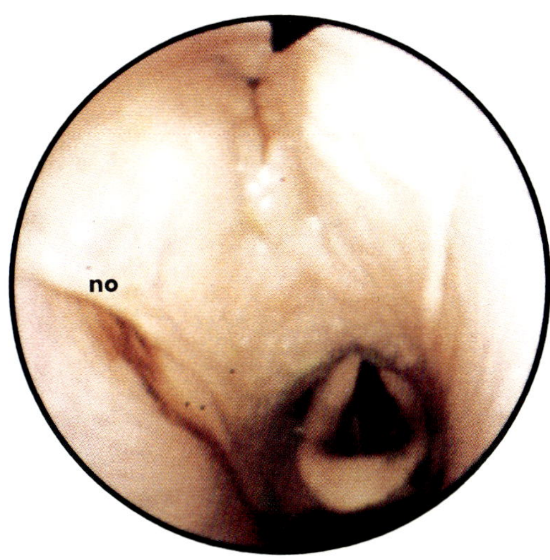

FIG. 5-16   Nasopharynx of a horse with guttural pouch mycosis. Note the serosanguineous discharge from the right nasopharyngeal orifice *(no)*.

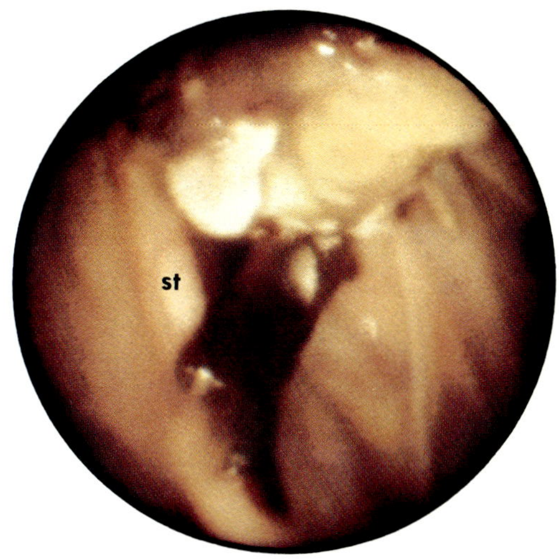

FIG. 5-17   Small mycotic plaque at the dorsocaudal extremity of the medial compartment of the right guttural pouch, adjacent to the insertion of the stylohyoid bone *(st)*.

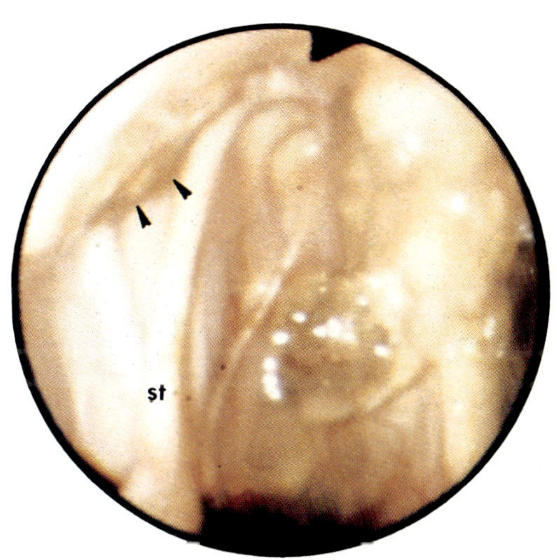

FIG. 5-18   Large pedunculated mycotic plaque in the medial compartment of the right guttural pouch. The mass limits visualization of the caudomedial portion of the medial compartment. A small plaque is also visible in the dorsal portion of the lateral compartment *(arrows)*. The tip of the endoscope is in the same location as in Fig. 5-7 *(st* indicates stylohyoid bone).

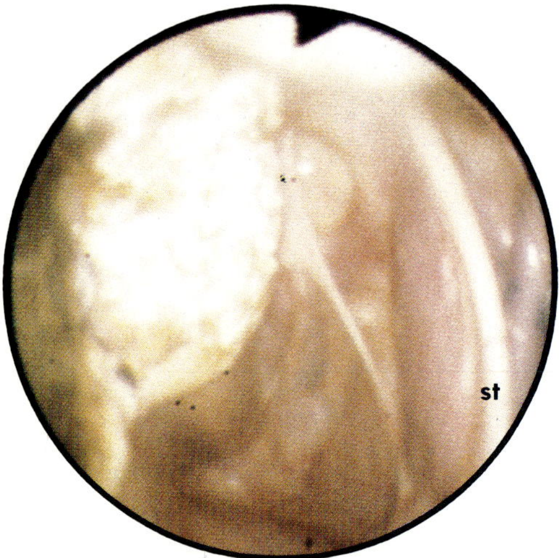

FIG. 5-19 Large mycotic plaque in
the left guttural pouch of the same horse
as in Fig. 5-18. The fungus had eroded
through the medial septum (*st* indicates
stylohyoid bone).

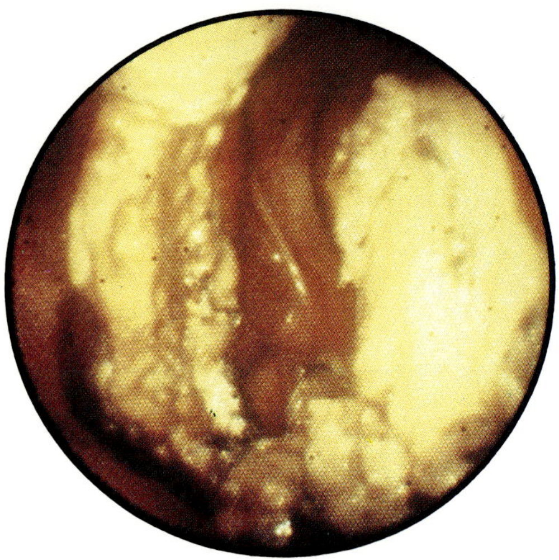

**FIG. 5-20 Close-up of mycotic
plaque** surrounding the internal carotid
artery and adjacent cranial nerves.

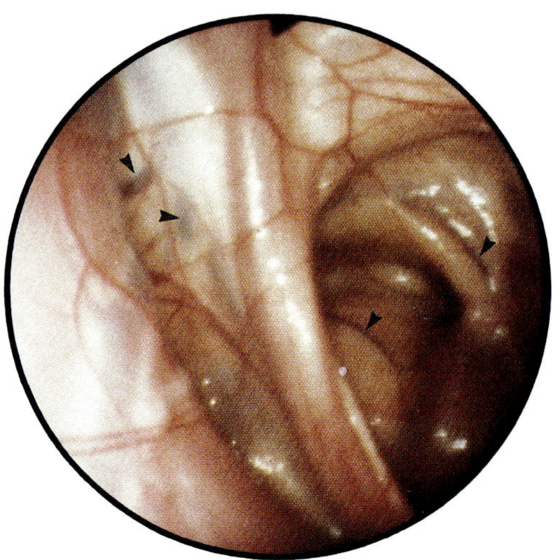

**FIG. 5-21 Interior of the guttural
pouch** of a horse with parotid
melanomata. Lymphatic vessels filled
with neoplastic cells are visible in
various locations *(arrows)*. (The intensity
of the black color has been decreased in
photograph preparation.)

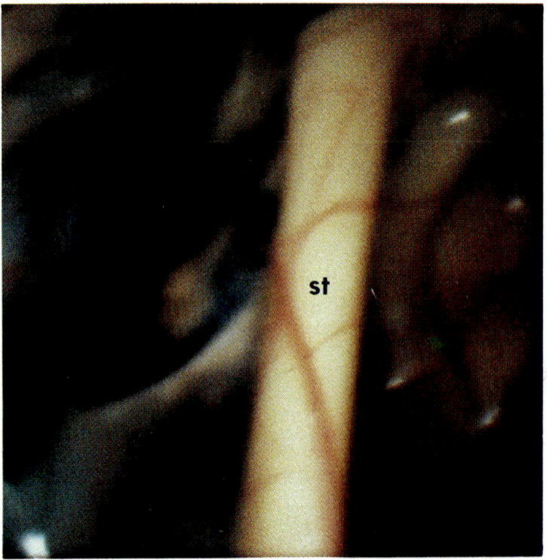

FIG. 5-22 Guttural pouch of a horse
with melanoma of the adjacent tissues.
Pigmented masses are visible through
the mucosa of the medial compartment,
to the left of the stylohyoid bone *(st)*.

TABLE 5-1 Guttural pouch diseases

CONDITION	CLINICAL SIGNS
Empyema (Figs. 5-13 thru 5-15)	Unilateral nasal discharge; parotid swelling; discharge from nasopharygeal orifice of affected pouch; "Chondroids" in chronic cases.
Mycosis (Figs. 5-16 thru 5-20)	Profuse epistaxis; neurologic signs referable to cranial nerve damage; serosanguineous/sanguineous discharge from nasopharyngeal orifice; mycotic plaque(s) in the affected pouch.
Tympany	External swelling of parotid/throatlatch region; attenuation of the nasopharyngeal lumen; occasionally accompanied by bacterial infection (empyema).
Neoplasia (Figs. 5-21 and 5-22)	Endoscopic abnormalities; depends on extent and type of tumor.

caudal wall of the medial compartment. It is easily identified by the pulsation of the internal carotid artery. The nerves and artery are closely apposed at the dorsal portion of the medial compartment but diverge distally. The nature of this divergence varies among individuals (Fig. 5-10 and 5-11). The pharyngeal branches of the vagus nerve and the cranial laryngeal nerve are often visible through the floor mucosa of the medial compartment, and the medial retropharyngeal lymph nodes are also related to the floor in this area (Fig. 5-12). The latter are not normally seen as distinct structures but invaginate the floor of the lateral and ventral portions of the medial compartment.

The right and left guttural pouches are separated dorsally by the *rectus capitus ventralis* and *longus capitus* muscles and cranioventrally by a medial septum comprising the fused mucosal walls of the opposing medial compartments (Fig 5-12). Both the lateral and the medial compartments are related to several important neural, vascular, and lymphatic structures. These structures are located outside the pouch lumen but can be seen through the translucent mucous membrane.

Table 5-1 includes guttural pouch diseases (Figs. 5-13 through 5-22).

Chapter 6

LARYNX

PETER F. HAYNES

The larynx is a dynamic upper respiratory tract (URT) structure, critically located between the nasopharynx and oropharynx and the trachea. Whereas normal laryngeal function is to protect the lower respiratory tract from contamination by ingesta, abnormal laryngeal function is most frequently characterized by signs referable to the respiratory system. Most disorders of the larynx do not affect the sedentary horse; however, optimal laryngeal function is vital to horses involved in strenuous athletic activity.

Diseases of the equine larynx are the single most frequent cause of upper respiratory obstructive disease. Therefore, it is imperative that the equine clinician examining the URT know the endoscopic anatomy and function of the larynx, whether examining a patient during a purchase examination or in response to complaints of exercise intolerance or abnormal respiratory noise.

This chapter describes considerations in the technique of endoscopic examination of the larynx and will review the pertinent anatomical and functional details of laryngeal assessment.

TECHNIQUE

Endoscopic evaluation of the larynx is routinely performed via the nasal cavity with the horse *at rest*. The endoscope is introduced through the ventral nasal meatus, and the field of view of the larynx is established on entry to the caudal nasopharynx.

The usual restraint employed for endoscopy of the larynx is a lip twitch. Patients resisting routine restraint for endoscopy may require chemical restraint to facilitate a thorough endoscopic evaluation of the URT to protect the patient, endoscopist, and instruments. Use of chemical restraints, including acepromazine maleate, xylazine, or combinations thereof, is controversial because it may change (reduce) abductor function (opening or dilation) of the arytenoid cartilages.[10,11] However, studies are not available to either validate or negate this concern.

Evaluation of laryngeal function, particularly *abductor* function, in patients intolerant of exercise and/or having abnormal respiratory noise is critical. If routine endoscopic examination fails to demonstrate appropriate abductor function, dynamic laryngeal activity may be induced in the patient at rest by the following techniques.

Induced swallow reflex. The swallow reflex is most conveniently induced by the administration of water through the flushing channel of the flexible fiberoptic endoscope. Instillation of 3 to 5ml into the nasopharynx will usually be followed by a swallow. With the overall view of the larynx maintained, near-maximum abduction of the arytenoid cartilages can be observed following this maneuver. Alternatives to water instillation include direct contact of the endoscope tip with the caudal soft palate or epiglottis.

Nasal occlusion. Air deprivation by nasal occlusion during endoscopy will induce spontaneous arytenoid movements, including laryngeal adduction (constriction or closure) and near-maximum abduction. The clinician must be aware that if use of this technique is prolonged, air hunger will cause the patient to become quite apprehensive or violent.

Slap test. This technique will induce arytenoid adduction in patients with intact spinal reflexes.[4] A crisp slap to the caudoventral hollow of the withers should induce arytenoid adduction on the contralateral side of the larynx. My experience indicates that in apprehensive patients that maintain arytenoid abduction, the slap test may not be effective. Additionally, adduction of the ipsilateral arytenoid frequently occurs but to a lesser extent than the contralateral cartilage.

Chemical induction. Doxapram is a respiratory stimulant used by some clinicians to facilitate evaluation of laryngeal abductor function.[11] Its effectiveness has not been reported.

Rebreathing. A 20 to 30 L plastic bag secured to the patient's facial region will drive respiration by forcing the patient to rebreathe increased carbon dioxide concentrations. An endoscope introduced through a portal in the bag and positioned in the caudal nasopharynx will allow observation of increased laryngeal activity.

Endoscopic evaluation of laryngeal function *after exercise* provides an excellent perspective of spontaneously induced laryngeal activity. It reflects the patient's natural response to an increased rate and volume of airflow through the respiratory conduit. The patient should be exercised until it has a respiratory rate of at least 80 to 100 breaths per minute. This allows the endoscopist 1 to 2 minutes to restrain the patient and observe spontaneous maximum or near-maximum arytenoid abduction.

Additional techniques

Additional techniques for endoscopic characterization of the laryngeal cartilages and/or laryngeal function will depend on the disorder observed, the endoscopic instrumentation available, and the exercise facilities used. These techniques include the following.

Endoscopy per os.   This technique is indicated for patients with a short epiglottis that cannot be observed by nasopharyngeal endoscopy (Fig. 6-1).[5] Endoscopy *per os* must be conducted with the patient under general anesthesia to protect the endoscope from being bitten. A mouth wedge is inserted to open the oral cavity, and a short endotracheal tube is inserted to the level of the caudal oropharynx. A Cole endotracheal tube is appropriate, though any relatively rigid tube 18 to 20 inches long that will allow unrestricted passage of the endoscope is adequate. Insertion of this endoscopic cannula should displace the soft palate dorsal to the epiglottis and allow full view of the epiglottis caudal to the base of the tongue.

Retrotracheal endoscopy.   Retrotracheal evaluation of the larynx is indicated for patients with extreme laryngeal obstruction (e.g. severe edema or inflammation, or distortion secondary to arytenoid chondritis) that precludes characterization of the laryngeal lumen by routine nasopharyngeal endoscopy. Because patients with such laryngeal obstruction are usually dyspneic at rest and require a tracheostomy, the clinician may perform retrograde endoscopic examination of the larynx through that portal. *Direct laryngeal endoscopy* may be performed after surgery in patients with a ventral laryngotomy to assess healing of operative sites within the larynx.

Video endoscopic evaluation during exercise.   The recent availability of video endoscopes has enhanced the opportunity to examine the "stationary" patient during exercise on a high-speed treadmill. Video endoscopy allows convenient viewing on a video monitor (rather than through the endoscope eyepiece) and should provide definitive characterization of many dynamic URT obstructive disorders, including laryngeal disease in athletic horses.

In completing the discussion of laryngeal evaluation, it is important to emphasize that observations should be documented (e.g., on

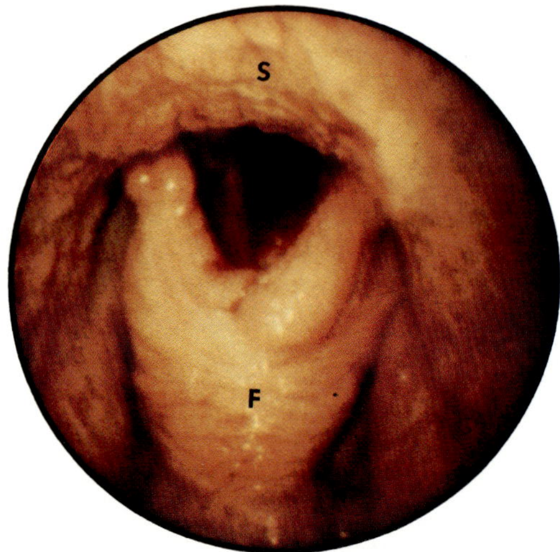

FIG. 6-1 Epiglottic shortening. Endoscopic view of a short epiglottis visualized during endoscopy *per os*. Nasopharyngeal endoscopy had revealed persistent dorsal displacement of the soft palate. The soft palate *(S)* is in the dorsal field of view and the rostral portion of the epiglottis is absent. The glossoepiglottic fold *(F)* is readily apparent. (Refer to Fig. 6-2D for further anatomical orientation.)

(From Haynes PF: Surgery of the respiratory tract. In Jennings Jr PB, editor: Practice of large animal surgery, Philadelphia, 1984, WB Saunders Co.)

medical records and by photography when available). Endoscopic examination of the URT is indicated for patients with substantiated clinical signs or for patients with a history suggesting a URT disorder. The endoscopist may need to perform sequential examinations to determine the presence, progression, or resolution of variations from normal laryngeal function. Additionally, because legal challenges to endoscopic opinions or diagnoses (specifically concerning the purchase examination) have become more common and accurate, complete documentation of observations will support the endoscopist's diagnosis.

ANATOMY AND FUNCTION

The general objectives of endoscopic examination of the URT are particularly important in evaluating the larynx and include assessment of the shape and size of laryngeal cartilages, the location and function (i.e., motion) of these cartilages, and the identification of any abnormal fluids, such as exudate or hemorrhage.

Anatomy

Fig. 6-2 demonstrates the anatomy of the larynx during nasopharyngeal endoscopy. Three laryngeal cartilages protrude rostrally through the intrapharyngeal ostium and are readily apparent during nasopharyngeal endoscopy: the paired corniculate cartilages (rostral extensions of the arytenoid cartilages) and the epiglottis. The *auditus laryngis* or pharyngeal opening of the larynx is bordered ventrally by the epiglottis, laterally by the aryepiglottic folds, and dorsally by the corniculate cartilages. The rima glottidis is the narrowest part of the laryngeal cavity and is bordered laterally by the vocal folds and dorsally by the axial surface of the arytenoid cartilages.[12] While the paired rostral cartilages of the larynx (which form the inverted V observed endoscopically) are frequently referred to as the arytenoid cartilages, they are actually the corniculate cartilages (corniculate processes of the arytenoid cartilages) composed of elastic cartilage, in contrast to the hyaline arytenoid cartilages of which they are an extension.* The mucosal surface of the corniculate cartilages is characterized by numerous small lymphoid aggregations, giving them a "pimpled" appearance.

The paired vocal folds (cords) are readily evident within the laryngeal lumen and form the V-shaped appearance in the rima glot-

---

*Hereafter, *corniculate* cartilages will be used in reference to that aspect of the arytenoid apparatus readily visible in the caudal nasopharynx. When referring to abduction or adduction, the term *arytenoid* will be used, understanding that any movement of the corniculate cartilages is a function of the intrinsic musculature attached to the arytenoid cartilages.

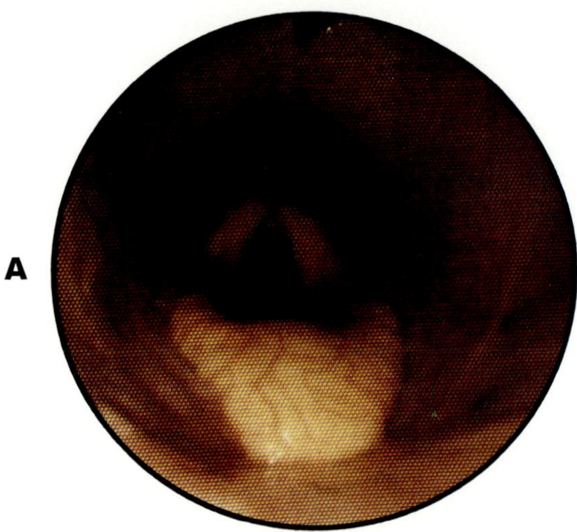

FIG. 6-2 **Endoscopic anatomy of the larynx. A, Overview of the larynx.** This view was obtained from the mid-nasopharyngeal region and is intended to demonstrate the normal position and appearance of the epiglottis. Note the serrated margin of the epiglottis and its dorsal vascular pattern. The paired corniculate cartilages are evident in the background. **B,** Close-up view of larynx. This view was obtained from just above the epiglottic apex and shows the corniculate cartilages in the resting or paramedian position.

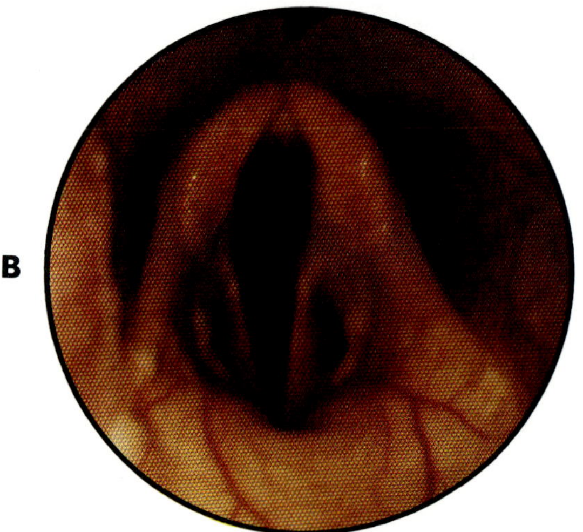

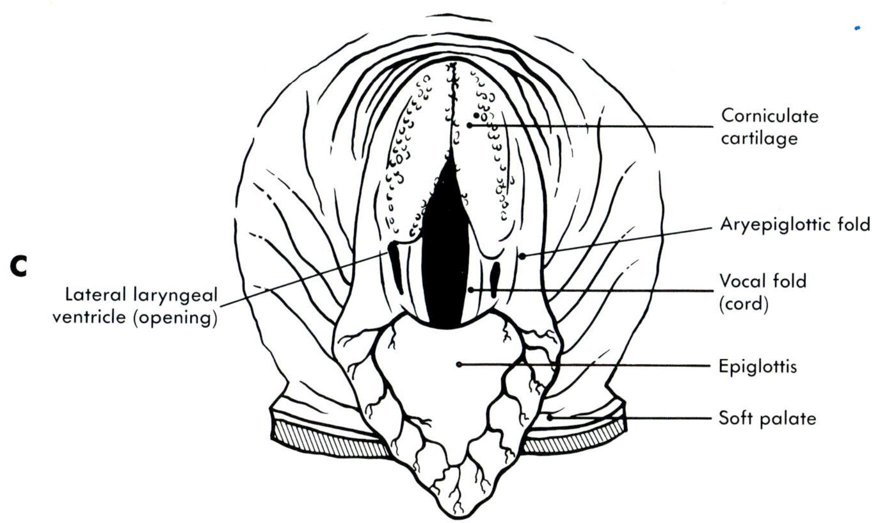

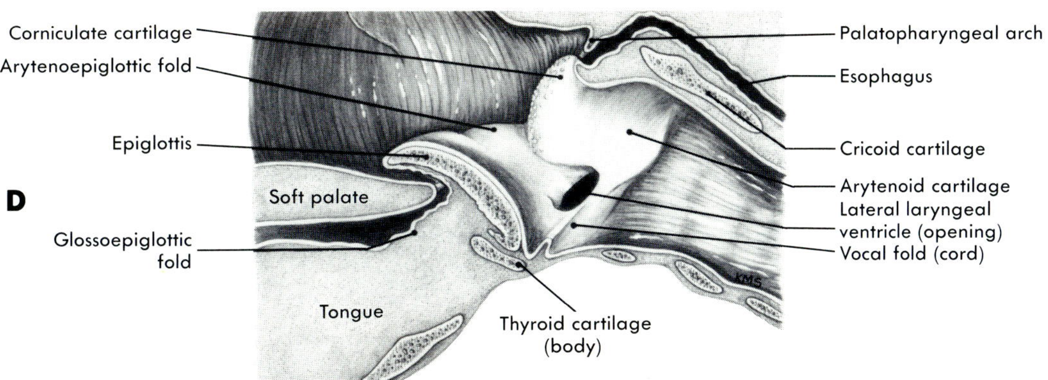

C, Diagrammatic representation of laryngeal anatomy, frontal view. This diagram is a composite of the laryngeal anatomy seen in the endoscopic views shown in **A** and **B.** **D,** Diagrammatic representation of laryngeal anatomy, saggital view. The diagram provides a spatial perspective of the laryngeal structures not fully appreciated in the frontal view.

(**C** and **D** from: Haynes PF: Surgery of the respiratory tract. In: Jennings Jr PB, editor: Practice of large animal surgery, Philadelphia, 1984, WB Saunders Co.)

tidis and extend dorsolaterally. The openings of the lateral laryngeal ventricles are apparent as indentations on the rostrolateral aspect of the vocal folds.

The elastic, epiglottic cartilage extends into the ventral nasopharynx and usually lies in contact with the soft palate below. The epiglottis is leaf shaped, being widest as it protrudes through the intrapharyngeal ostium and narrowing to a rostral apex. The convex dorsal surface is covered with a smooth and glistening respiratory mucosa that exposes a vascular pattern along its serrated margins. The aryepiglottic fold is the mucosal "sling" for the epiglottis and is endoscopically seen as a fold of tissue extending from the ventrolateral aspect of each corniculate cartilage to the caudolateral margin of the epiglottis.

In patients with an axially displaced corniculate cartilage (e.g., arytenoid chondritis), the palatopharyngeal fold may become evident on that side (Fig. 6-5, *C*). This rim of tissue is the lateral aspect of the intrapharyngeal ostium, which separates the oropharynx from the nasopharynx and extends dorsally, becoming confluent with its contralateral part as the palatopharyngeal arch (Fig. 6-3, and see Fig. 6-5, *B*, p. 69). In patients with normal pharyngeal and laryngeal function, the margin of the intrapharyngeal ostium is constricted about the posterior aspect of the epiglottic and corniculate cartilages and is not evident endoscopically.

Definitive assessment of the epiglottis may require endoscopy *per os* when the epiglottis is not seen during nasopharyngeal endoscopy (e.g., persistent dorsal displacement of the soft palate secondary to a short epiglottis) (Fig. 6-1).[5] During oral endoscopy, as described earlier, dorsal displacement of the soft palate occurs in such a way that the epiglottis and subepiglottic tissues should be readily apparent. The epiglottis is located above the glossoepiglottic fold, which is a continuum of mucosa between the epiglottis and the caudal tongue. The appearance of the epiglottis should resemble one seen during nasopharyngeal endoscopy, with the exception that the epiglottis will have a greater ventral curvature because of its lack of ventral soft palate support (Fig. 4-4, *D*, p. 36).

Function

Endoscopic evaluation of laryngeal function is of paramount importance in the diagnosis of the most common laryngeal diseases, including idiopathic laryngeal hemiplegia (Fig. 6-4), arytenoid chondritis (Fig. 6-5) and epiglottic entrapment (Fig. 6-6).[7] Although arytenoid adduction acts to protect the lower respiratory tract from ingesta, loss of this function is seldom of clinical importance. However, loss of arytenoid abduction is critical in horses expected to perform most athletic activities. Thus it is imperative to allow adequate time during examination to fully assess laryngeal function,

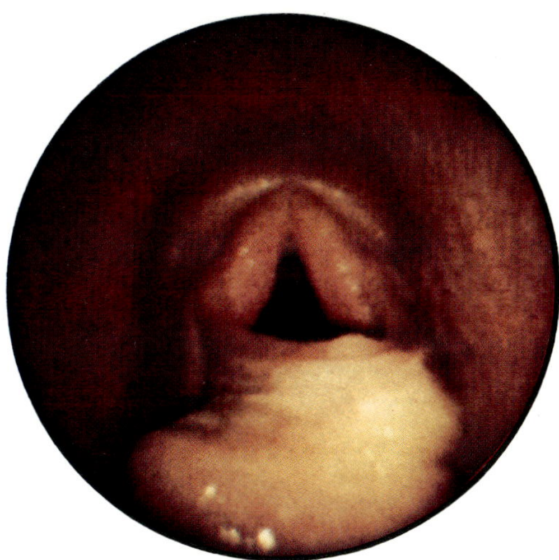

FIG. 6-3 Subepiglottic cyst. Endoscopic view demonstrating a subepiglottic cyst lying on the floor of the nasopharynx. The cyst, which occasionally disappeared from view (relocating in the oropharynx), markedly elevated the apex of the epiglottis when in this nasopharyngeal position. (NOTE: The palatopharyngeal arch is more evident above the corniculate cartilages than usual, though this occasional observation during endoscopy is an acceptable variation of normal.)

(From Haynes PV: Surgery of the respiratory tract. In: Jennings Jr PB, editor: Practice of large animal surgery, Philadelphia, 1984, WB Saunders Co.)

particularly arytenoid abduction.

Appreciation of laryngeal function (as well as the size and shape of its cartilages) is based on the premise that the larynx is symmetric from one side to the other; thus the larynx must be viewed from a position directly ahead of it. If the endoscopist believes that symmetry may be biased by a diagonal view, an effort should be made to appropriately redirect the tip of the endoscope. Furthermore, the endoscope may be reinserted through the contralateral nasal cavity to determine if an impression of asymmetry is real or artifactual. Because some patients exhibit little spontaneous arytenoid movement, it may be appropriate to induce motion as described previously.

Three basic positions of the arytenoid apparatus are recognized: fully adducted (closed), resting (paramedian), and fully abducted (open) (Fig. 6-7 and Fig. 6-2).[2] While normal arytenoid movements in the resting horse may range from complete adduction to abduction, the arytenoids are usually paramedian. Spontaneous arytenoid movements should be synchronous with respiration (abduction during inspiration) and are usually characterized by submaximum abduction followed by a return to the paramedian position. Asynchronous abduction of the arytenoids may be an acceptable variation in 40% to 50% of the thoroughbred population[1,9] and is char-

Text continued on p. 72.

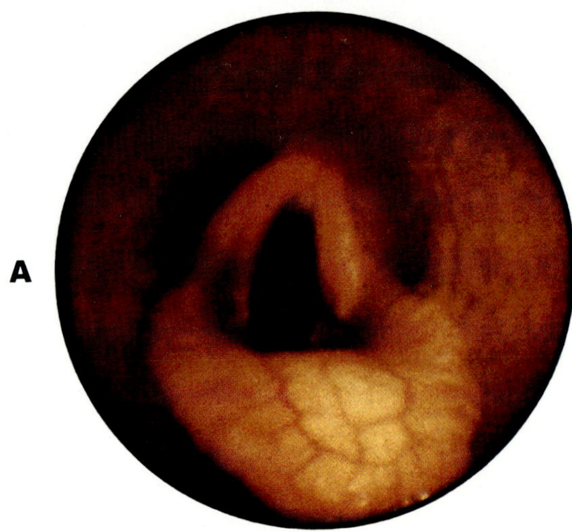

FIG. 6-4 Idiopathic laryngeal hemiplegia. A, Endoscopic view demonstrating the left corniculate cartilage in a paramedian position. The right corniculate cartilage is partially abducted, creating the asymmetry that is typical of this disease (NOTE: Observing the *active* abductor function of the larynx is critical in establishing this diagnosis.) **B,** Endoscopic view demonstrating lateralization of the left arytenoid apparatus following prosthetic laryngoplasty. The right corniculate cartilage is in a paramedian position. Adduction of the left arytenoid apparatus will not occur while it remains fixed in an abducted position.

(A from: Haynes PF: Surgery of the respiratory tract. In: Jennings Jr PB, editor: Practice of large animal surgery, Philadelphia, 1984, WB Saunders Co.)

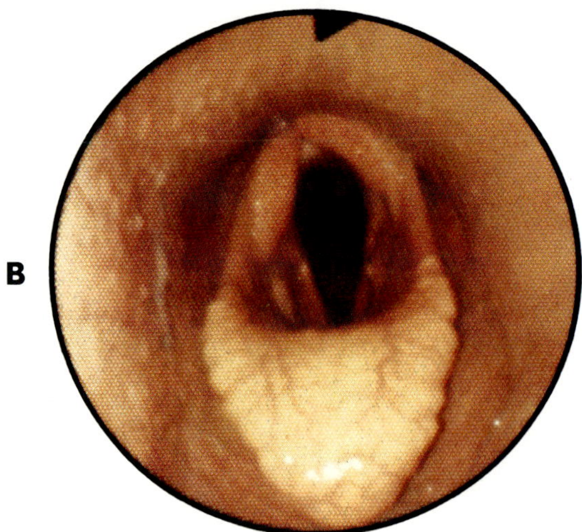

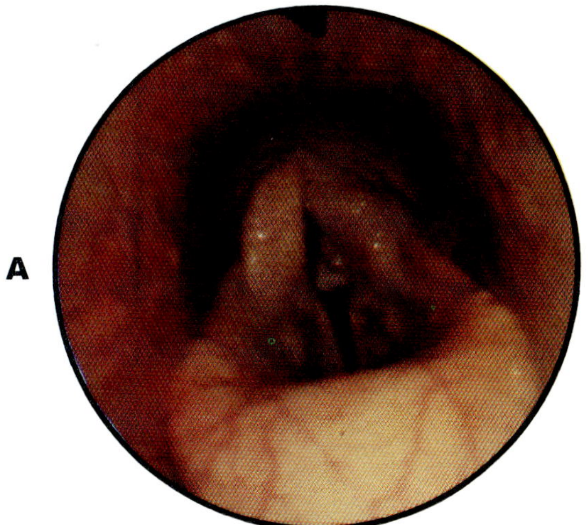

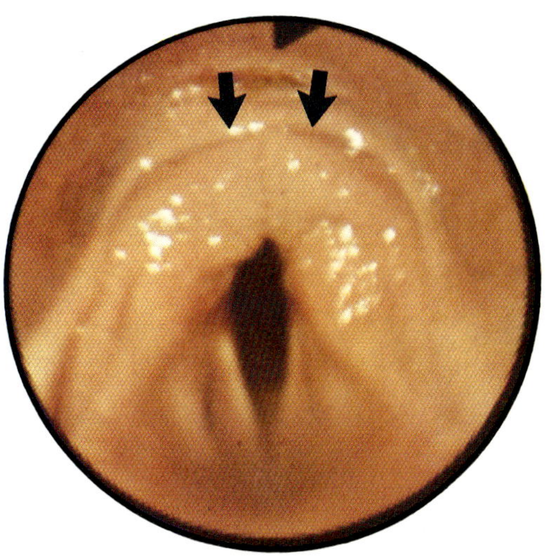

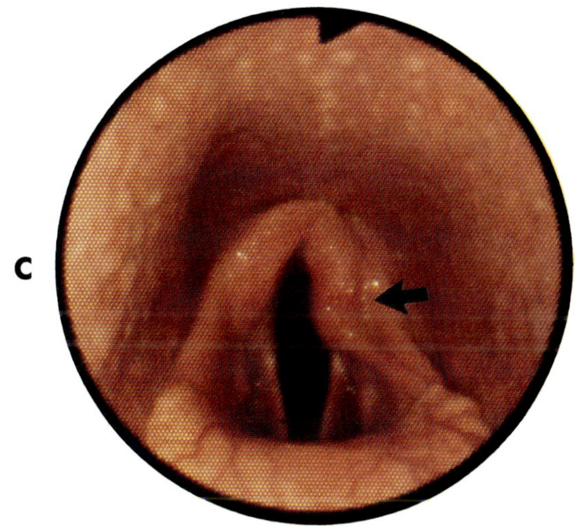

FIG. 6-5 Arytenoid chondritis. A, Endoscopic view demonstrating left arytenoid chondritis. Distortion of the left corniculate cartilage, a projection from the involved arytenoid cartilage into the laryngeal lumen and reduced abductor ability of the left hemilarynx confirmed the diagnosis in this patient. **B,** Endoscopic view demonstrating left arytenoid chondritis and perilaryngitis. Mucosal edema and inflammation of both the corniculate cartilages and palatopharyngeal arch, the slightly more axial position of the left corniculate cartilage and reduced abductor ability of the left hemilarynx contributed to the tenative diagnosis. The palatopharyngeal arch *(arrows)* is quite prominent and has a dorsal ulcer. (NOTE: After 30 days of treatment, re-examination revealed a larynx quite similar to that in A.) **C,** Endoscopic view demonstrating left arytenoid chondritis. The original diagnosis was left laryngeal hemiplegia. The near midline displacement of the left corniculate and the attending mucosal distortion lateral to it *(arrow)* contributed to the tentative diagnosis of arytenoid chondritis subsequently confirmed during surgery. (NOTE: The palatopharyngeal fold is evident on the left side.)

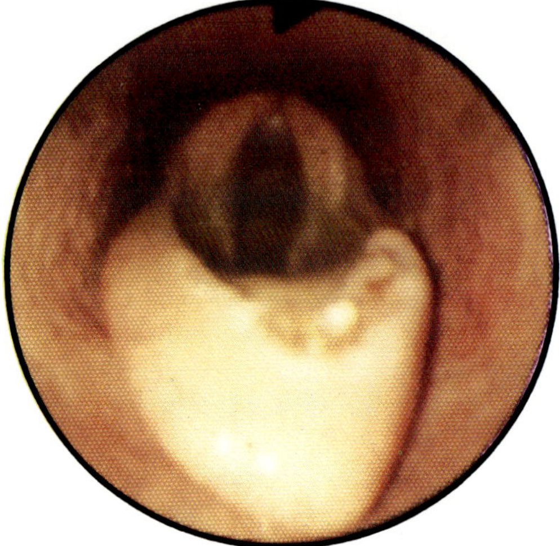

FIG. 6-6 Epiglottic entrapment. Endoscopic view demonstrating epiglottic entrapment with ulceration of the free margin of entrapping tissue on the left side. The profile of the epiglottis is apparent though its dorsal surface and margins are obscured from visualization by the subepiglottic mucosa enveloping it. (NOTE: This condition must be distinguished from dorsal displacement of the soft palate since a free margin of tissue just rostral to the auditus laryngis is characteristic of both conditions. See Fig. 4-7B, p. 41.)

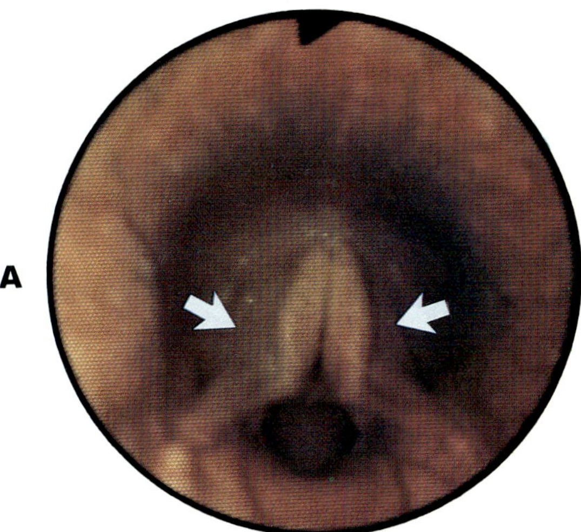

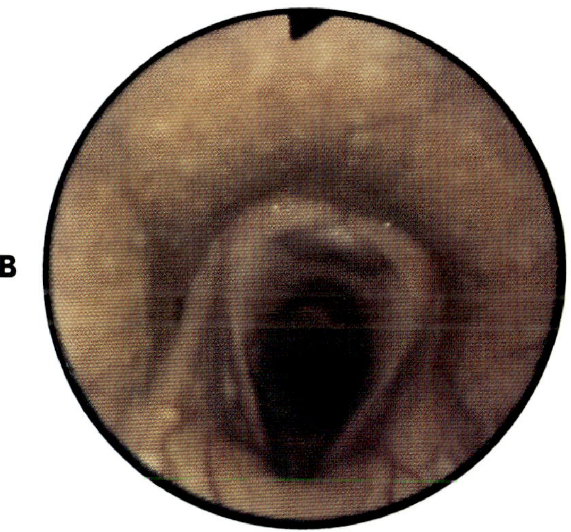

FIG. 6-7 Corniculate (arytenoid) positions. A, Endoscopic view of the fully adducted (constricted) larynx. The corniculate cartilages contact each other on the midline. With the larynx in adduction, the lateral margins of the intrapharyngeal ostium (palatopharyngeal folds) become more evident *(arrows)*. **B,** Endoscopic view of the fully abducted (dilated) larynx. The corniculate cartilages are rotated dorsolaterally and contact the roof of the nasopharynx.

TABLE 6-1 Diseases of the larynx

DISEASE	CLINICAL SIGNS
1. Idiopathic laryngeal hemiplegia (hemiparesis)	Sustained exercise intolerance; inspiratory noise production
2. Arytenoid chondritis	Sustained exercise intolerance; inspiratory noise production, including dyspnea at rest in advanced cases
3. Epiglottic entrapment	Range from exercise intolerance and inspiratory/expiratory noise production to asymptomatic
4. Epiglottic shortening/ hypoplasia	Sustained exercise intolerance and abnormal noise production, compatible with persistent dorsal displacement of the soft palate
5. Epiglottic or subepiglottic ulceration	Sustained exercise intolerance; anorexia; dysphagia, coughing while eating
6. Subepiglottic cyst	Sustained exercise intolerance; abnormal noise production and coughing/dysphagia, particularly in the foal
7. Neoplasia, granulomatous disease	Range from sustained exercise intolerance and abnormal noise production to dyspnea at rest including serosanguineous to mucopurulent nasal discharge

acterized by delayed, biphasic or multiphasic abduction, usually in the left hemilarynx. In the patient examined at rest, complete adduction and abduction are usually apparent only following nasal occlusion and/or stimulation of the swallowing reflex, respectively. Observation of maximum abductor function in the left hemilarynx may reduce the concern of asynchronous arytenoid motion. Spontaneous, maximum arytenoid abduction can be observed most ideally with video endoscopy during treadmill exercise, or it may be apparent immediately following sustained exercise.

The characterization of reduced arytenoid adductor or abductor function may range from partial to complete. Reduction of arytenoid adductor function may support a diagnosis of idiopathic laryngeal hemiplegia or hemiparesis[3] and may also assist in identifying patients with fixed arytenoid abduction following a prosthetic laryngoplasty (Fig. 6-4, *A*). Reduction of arytenoid abductor function most frequently supports the diagnosis of idiopathic laryngeal hemiplegia, hemiparesis, or arytenoid chondritis. Although hemiplegia is predominantly a disease of the left hemilarynx, arytenoid chondritis affects both sides of the larynx with equal frequency.[8] The endoscopist should be familiar with the characteristics of each disease because they are frequently confused, particularly in cases of early arytenoid chondritis. A follow-up examination 3 to 4 weeks later may allow more precise characterization of the underlying problem.

While the arytenoid apparatus has deserved primary focus of laryngeal function based on morbidity, this section would be incomplete without comments on epiglottic function. Routine nasopharyngeal endoscopy should reveal the epiglottis in its normal nasopharyngeal (suprapalatal) position and allow characterization of its size and shape, including the presence of any abnormalities. However, in some patients, particularly those apprehensive to nasopharyngeal endoscopy and its attending restraint maneuvers, the epiglottis may not be visible. If the epiglottis is not observed, the endoscopist should stimulate one or more swallow reflexes and consider reducing restraint techniques (e.g., lip twitch). The epiglottis will usually resume its nasopharyngeal position unless it is abnormally short or otherwise restricted from its normal range of motion.[6,7] Such cases will require oral endoscopy (described earlier) to fully characterize the epiglottis.

Table 6-1 lists diseases of the larynx evident by endoscopic examination (listed in order of decreasing frequency based on my experience).

REFERENCES

1. Baker GJ: Laryngeal asynchrony in the horse—definition and significance, In Snow DH, Person SGB, and Rose RJ editors: Equine Exercise Physiology, Cambridge, 1983, Granta Publications.
2. Cook WR: Some observations on form and function of the equine upper airway in health and disease: II Larynx, Proc 27th Annu Conv Am Assoc Equine Pract, 393:1981.
3. Duncan ID and Griffiths IR: Pathological changes in equine laryngeal muscles and nerves, Proc 19th Annu Conv Am Assoc Equine Pract, 97:1973.
4. Greet TRC et al: The slap test for laryngeal adductory function in horses with suspected cervical spinal cord damage, Equine Vet J 12:127, 1980.
5. Haynes PF: Persistent dorsal displacement of the soft palate associated with epiglottic shortening in two horses, J Am Vet Med Assoc 179:677, 1981.
6. Haynes PF: Dorsal displacement of the soft palate and epiglottic entrapment: diagnosis, management and interrelationship. Comp Cont Ed 5:S379, 1983.
7. Haynes PF: Surgery of the equine respiratory tract. In Jennings PB editor: The practice of large animal surgery, vol. 1, Philadelphia, 1984, WB Saunders Co.
8. Haynes PF: McClure JR, and Watters JW: Subtotal arytenoidectomy in the horse: an update, Proc 30th Annu Conv Am Assoc Equine Pract, 21, 1984.
9. Hillige CJ: Interpretation of laryngeal function tests in the horse, Vet Rec 118:535, 1986.

10. Koch C: Diseases of the larynx and pharynx of the horse, Comp Cont Ed 2(5):S73, 1980.
11. Lane JG: Fibreoptic endoscopy of the equine upper respiratory tract: a commentary on progress, Equine Vet J 196:495, 1987.
12. Sisson S and Grossman DR: The anatomy of the domestic animals, ed 4, Philadelphia, 1953, WB Saunders Co.

Chapter 7

TRACHEA AND BRONCHI

FREDERIK J. DERKSEN

Tracheoscopy and bronchoscopy are useful diagnostic aids in the examination of horses with lower airway disease. This chapter describes the techniques of tracheoscopy and bronchoscopy, and the endoscopic anatomy of the airways. It also shows some of the abnormalities that may be found by using these techniques.

TECHNIQUE

Tracheoscopy and bronchoscopy are performed with the standing horse restrained in stocks. A twitch may be used to aid in the restraint. Administration of xylazine (0.5 mg/kg of body weight) not only provides chemical restraint but also reduces coughing associated with bronchoscopy. A fiberoptic endoscope is passed via a nostril, ventral nasal meatus, pharynx, and larynx into the proximal trachea (Fig. 7-1). Most normal horses allow this procedure without showing signs of discomfort. If the endoscope is 1 m long, only the proximal trachea can be examined. A scope 150 cm long or longer is required to perform bronchoscopy (Fig. 7-2). The endoscope is advanced toward the carina (Fig. 7-3). Coughing is usually not elicited until the endoscope reaches the carina and may be minimized by introducing approximately 5 ml of 2% lidocaine into the biopsy channel of the bronchoscope and spraying this solution so that it coats the carina and right and left principal bronchi.

Bronchoscopic examination should be performed systematically. Each of the major bronchi should be examined in turn so that focal lesions in the airways are not missed. Using a 9 or 12 mm diameter endoscope, the clinician may enter all of the major bronchi and several of the segmental bronchi of the diaphragmatic lobe (Fig. 7-4).

75

Text continued on p. 78.

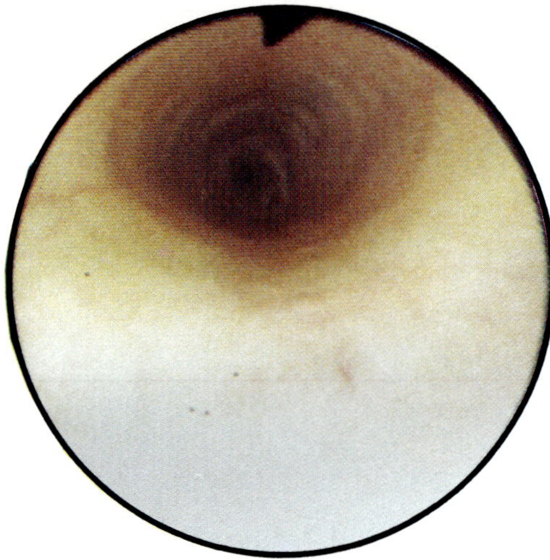

FIG. 7-1 The normal trachea.

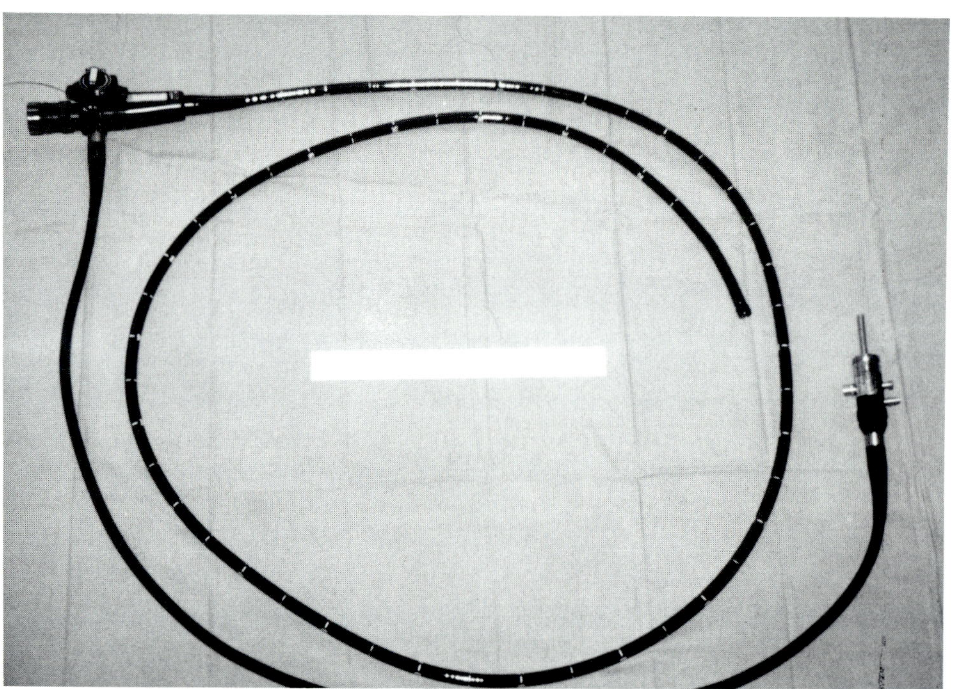

FIG. 7-2 Fiberoptic endoscope 3 m long, 12 mm diameter, used for bronchoscopy in the horse.

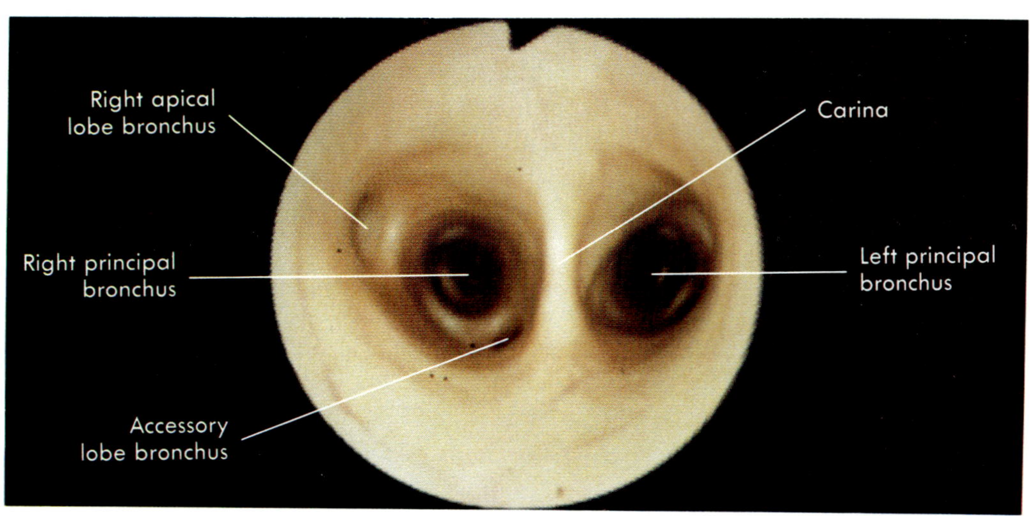

FIG. 7-3 The carina.

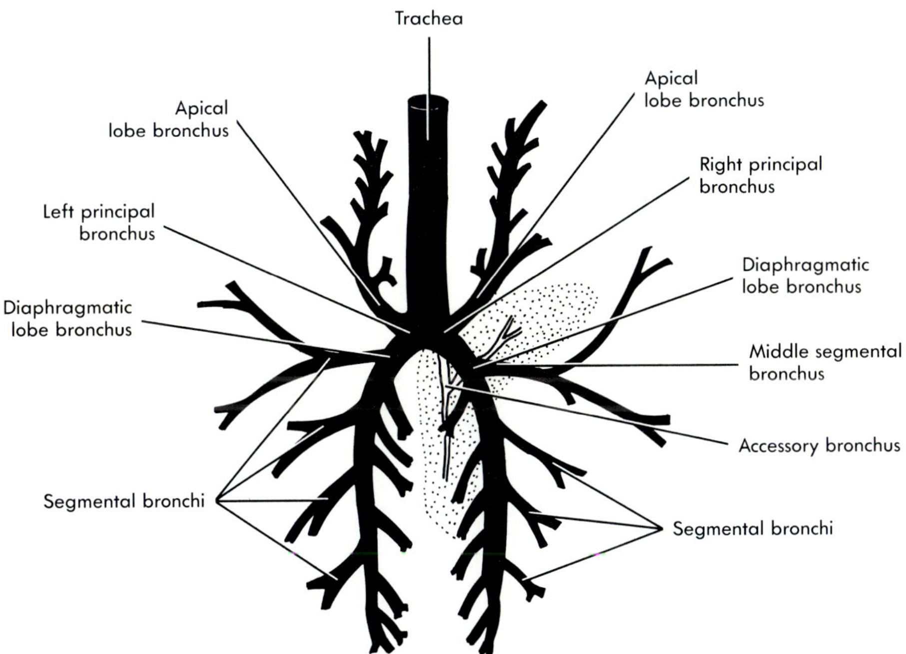

FIG. 7-4 Schematic dorsal view of the normal tracheobronchial tree.

ANATOMY

The trachea extends from the larynx to the carina, where it divides into the right and left principal bronchi. The trachea is approximately 75 to 80 cm long and has an average diameter of 5 to 6 cm. It is supported by 50 to 60 incomplete cartilaginous rings, the outline of which are easily discernible through the endoscope.

The right and left principal bronchi are formed by the bifurcation of the trachea approximately at the level of the fifth rib. The left principal bronchus is slightly smaller and makes a more acute angle with the trachea. As the right principal bronchus enters the lung, from its lateral aspect it gives off the apical lobar bronchus, which serves the apical lobe (Fig. 7-5). Further distally, the right principal bronchus gives off from its ventromedial aspect the accessory lobe bronchus, which ventilates the accessory lobe (Fig. 7-5). After giving off the accessory lobe bronchus, the principal bronchus continues caudally as the diaphragmatic lobe bronchus. The first segmental bronchus arises on the ventrolateral aspect and corresponds closely to the right middle lobe bronchus of other species. Therefore this bronchus is called the middle segmental bronchus (Fig. 7-6). After giving off the middle segmental bronchus, the right diaphragmatic lobe bronchus gives off several large segmental bronchi from its ventrolateral and dorsal aspects (Fig. 7-6). The branching pattern of the left principal bronchus is similar to that of the right except that the accessory lobe bronchus is absent in the left lung (Fig. 7-7).

Table 7-1 lists lower airway abnormalities (Figs. 7-8 through 7-17).

TABLE 7-1 Lower airway abnormalities that may be diagnosed endoscopically.

CONDITION	CLINICAL SIGNS
Trauma (Fig. 7-8)	Depends upon site and severity; may include epistaxis, coughing, dyspnea
Stricture (Fig. 7-9)	Slowly developing dyspnea, mostly inspiratory; exercise intolerance and sometimes cough
Chondroma (Fig. 7-10)	Depends upon the size—may be similar signs to stricture
Foreign body (Fig. 7-11)	Coughing; nasal discharge which may be hemorrhagic; malodorous breath
Hemorrhage (Fig. 7-12)	Most commonly due to exercise-induced pulmonary hemorrhage, associated with reduced performance and epistaxis
Purulent discharge (Fig. 7-13)	Coughing; nasal discharge; exercise intolerance; if septic, may be febrile
Pulmonary abscess (Fig. 7-14)	Coughing; nasal discharge which may be hemorrhagic; weight loss; fever; leucocytosis; may lead to pleuritis
Fungal infection (Fig. 7-15)	Coughing; nasal discharge; if severe, weight loss and exercise intolerance
Heart failure (Fig. 7-16)	Tachycardia, possibly arrhythmias or loud murmurs; jugular pulsation; peripheral edema; exercise intolerance
Tumor (Fig. 7-17)	Depends upon size and location; may have coughing; nasal discharge; dyspnea; weight loss

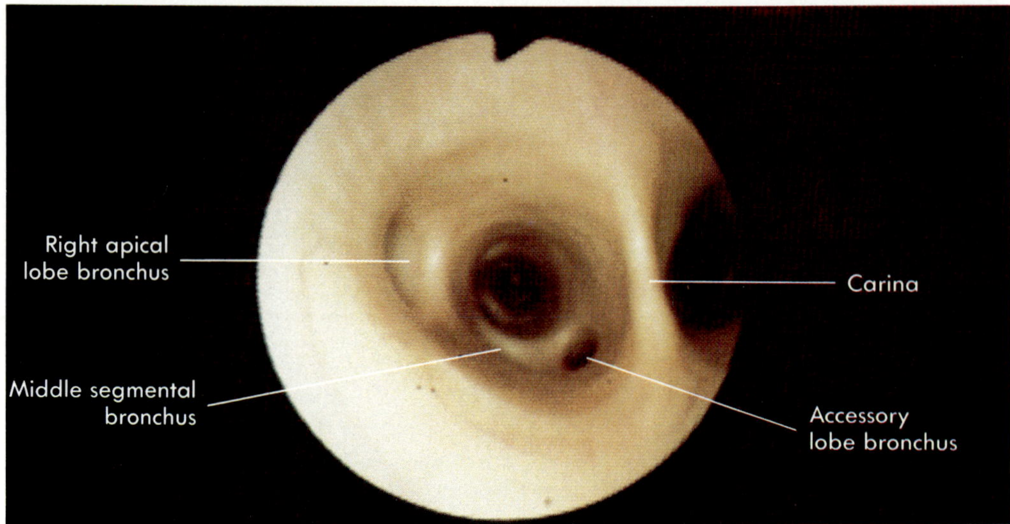

FIG. 7-5 The right principal bronchus. Note the apical lobe bronchus on the lateral aspect and the accessory lobe bronchus on the ventromedial aspect.

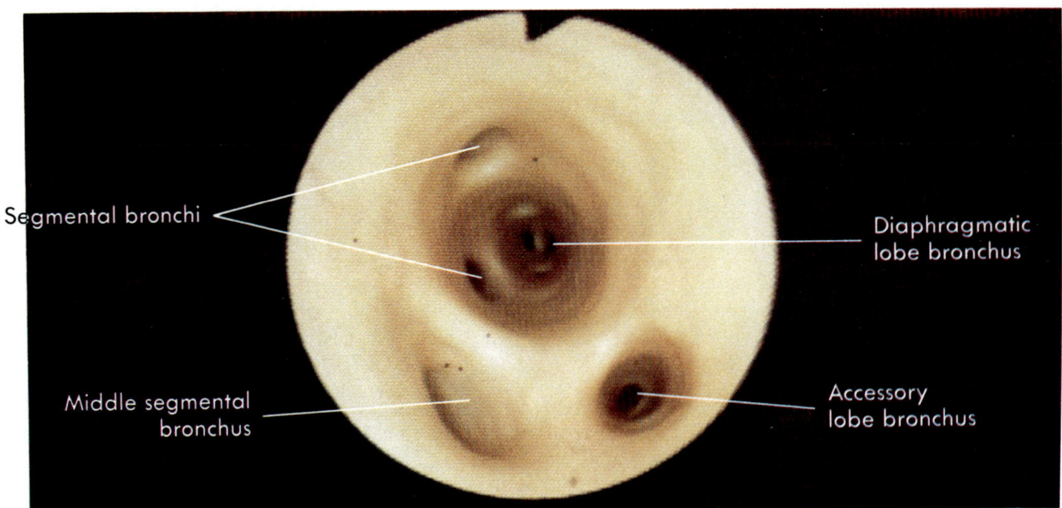

FIG. 7-6 The right principal and diaphragmatic lobe bronchi. Note the accessory lobe bronchus on the ventromedial aspect and the middle segmental bronchus on the ventrolateral aspect.

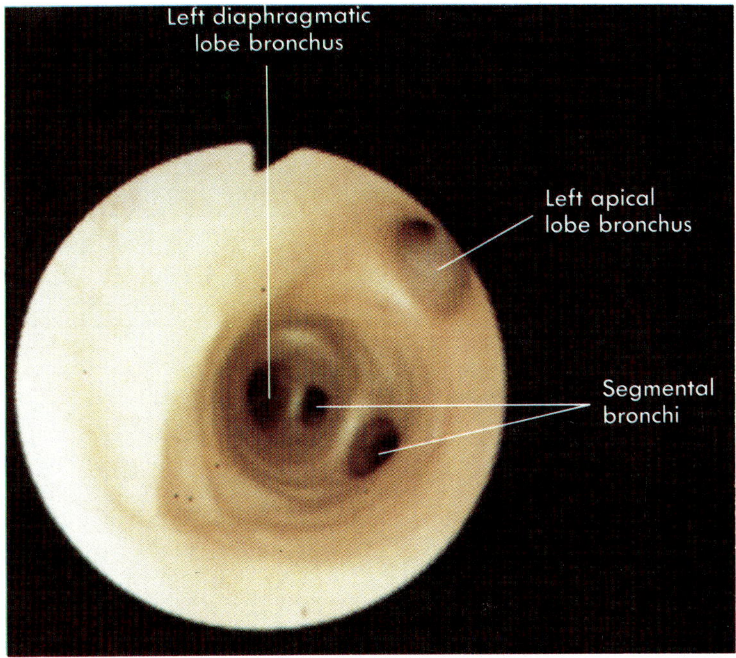

FIG. 7-7 The left principal and diaphragmatic lobe bronchi. Note the apical lobe bronchus on the dorsolateral aspect and the first segmental bronchus on the ventrolateral aspect.

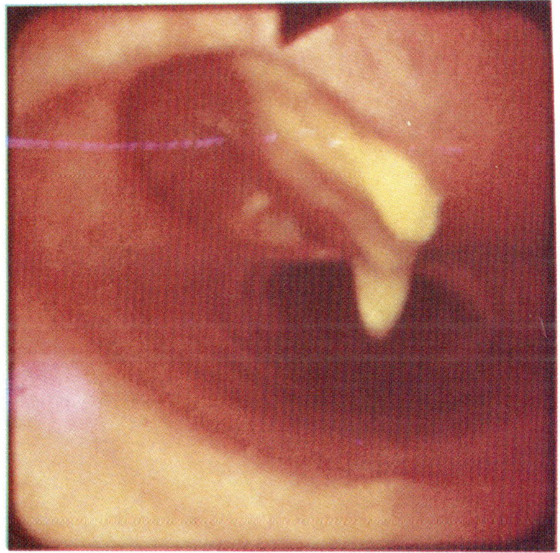

FIG. 7-8 Mucosal tear in the dorsal aspect of the midcervical trachea caused by blunt trauma.

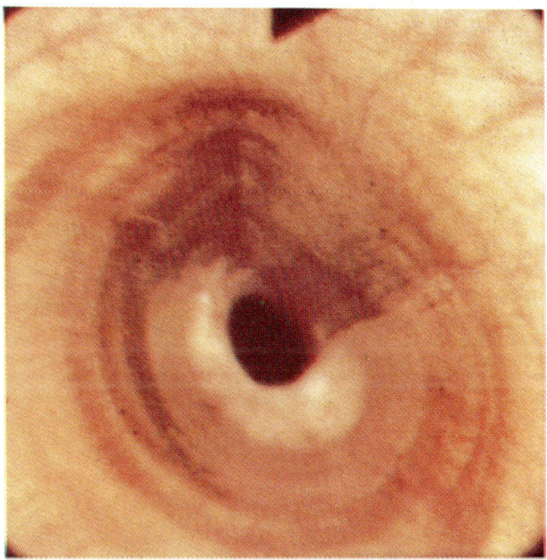

FIG. 7-9 Tracheal stricture formed after healing of blunt trauma.

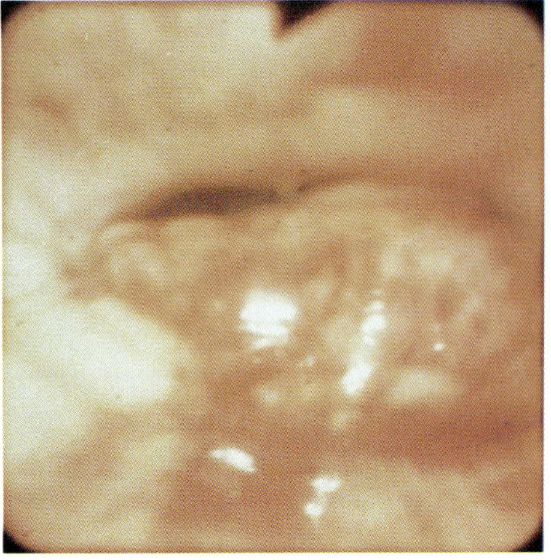

FIG. 7-10 **Tracheal chondroma** causing almost complete tracheal obstruction.

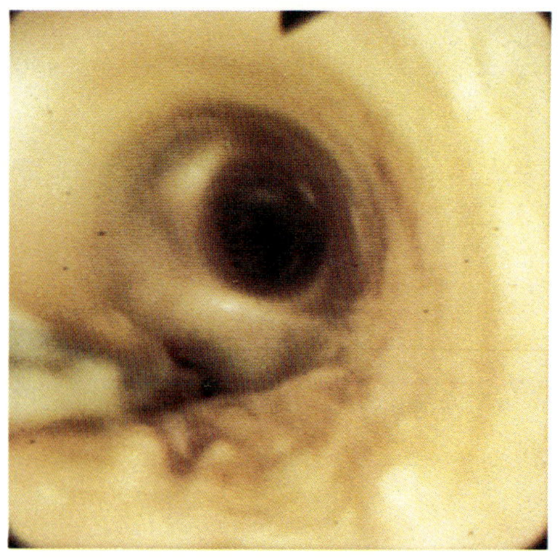

FIG. 7-11 **Thorned branch in the left principal bronchus** of a horse with a history of chronic coughing of several months duration.

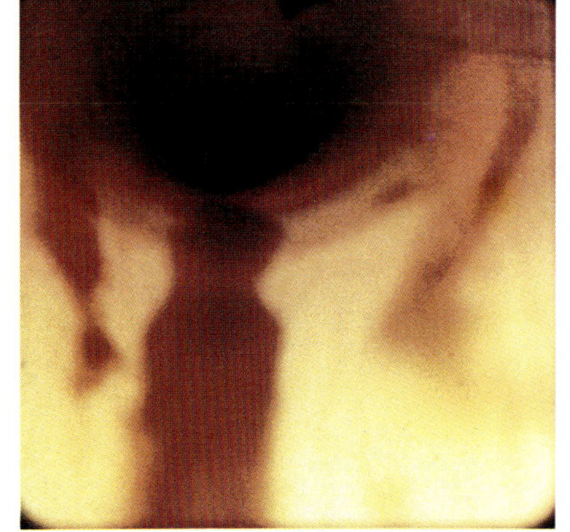

A

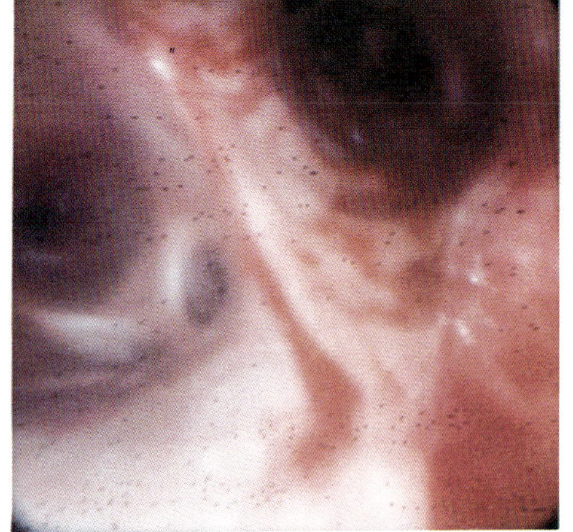

B

FIG. 7-12 **A, Exercise-induced pulmonary hemorrhage** in a 5-year-old Standardbred racehorse. **B,** Exercise-induced pulmonary hemorrhage from the left lung of a 7-year-old Standardbred. Photo was taken 15 minutes after exercise.

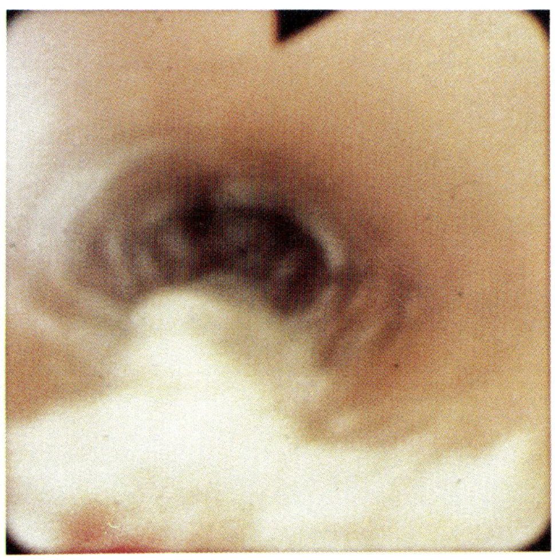

FIG. 7-13 Purulent tracheal discharge in a 12-year-old quarterhorse with chronic obstructive pulmonary disease.

A 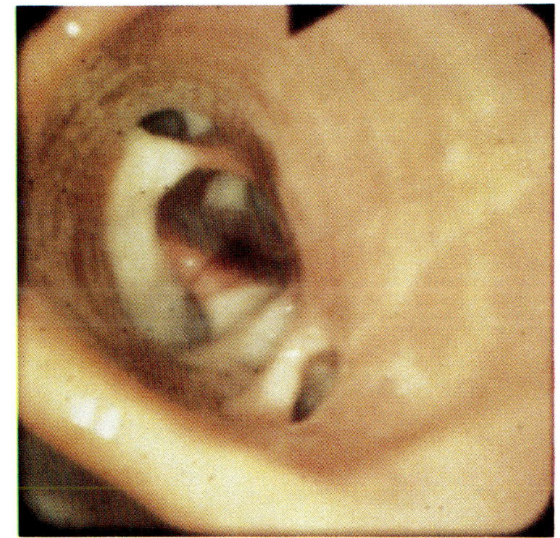 **B** 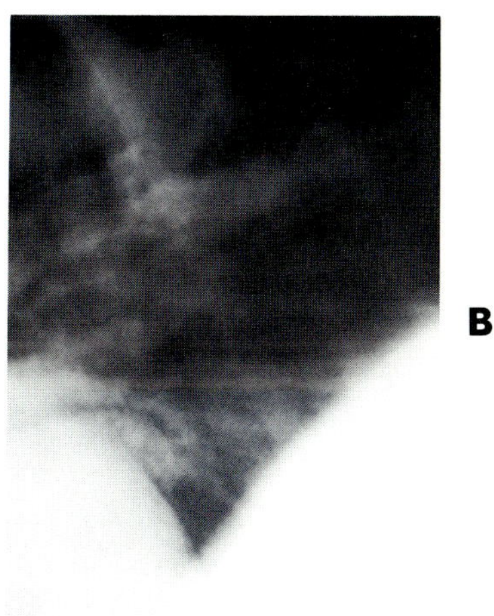

FIG. 7-14 Purulent discharge from a segmental bronchus in the diaphragmatic lobe **(A)** caused by a pulmonary abscess **(B).**

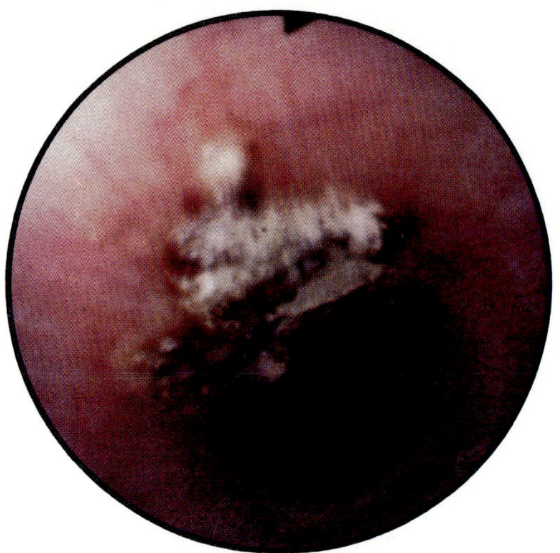

FIG. 7-15   Fungal tracheitis (*Aspergillus* spp) in a 3-week-old Percheron foal.

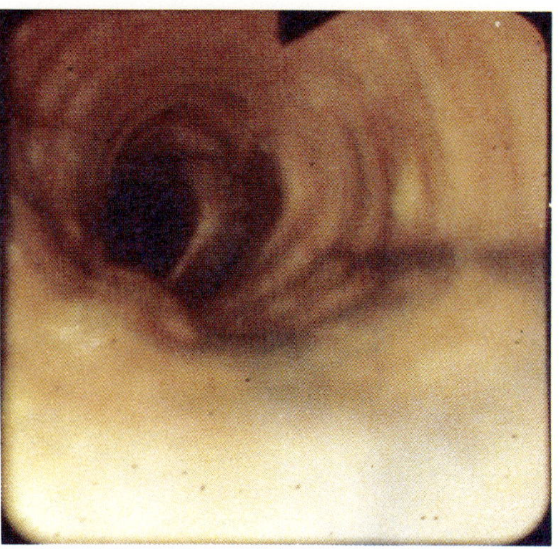

FIG. 7-16   Congestion of bronchial veins in a horse with heart failure.

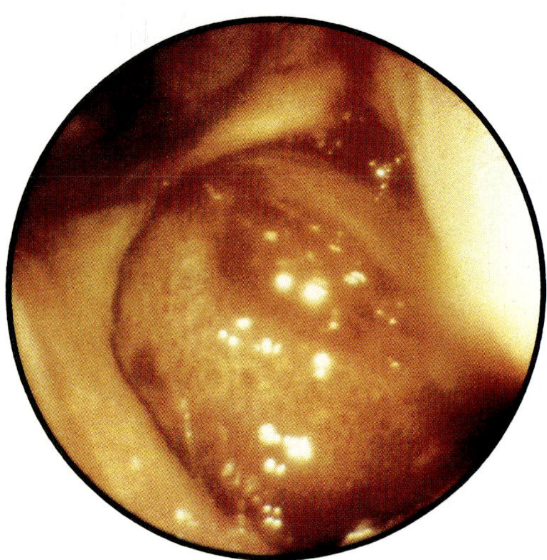

FIG. 7-17   Granular myoblastoma in the right principal bronchus of a 14-year-old Thoroughbred.

Chapter 8

TRANSENDOSCOPIC LASER SURGERY OF THE RESPIRATORY TRACT

ERIC P. TULLENERS

A laser is an electro-optical device capable of efficiently transmitting energy in the form of an intense, highly focused beam of light. *Laser* is an acronym for **L**ight **A**mplification by the **S**timulated **E**mission of **R**adiation. This is not ionizing radiation such as that produced by radiography. Properties of laser light that differ from incandescent light include (1) monochromaticity—the light emitted is of one or a few discrete wavelengths, (2) coherence—all wavelengths are in phase in time and space, and (3) collimation—all wavelengths are parallel, with very little beam divergence.

The radiant energy of the laser beam is transformed into thermal energy that produces the medical and surgical effects on tissue.[7] Possible interactions of the laser beam with tissue include reflection, scattering, transmission, and absorption. The three medically important lasers currently in common use are the carbon dioxide (CO_2), argon, and neodymium:yttrium aluminum and garnet (neodymium:YAG) lasers, which are named after the lasing medium used.

Factors influencing tissue effects include power or energy density, spot size, and the spectral absorption characteristics of the tissue irradiated. Laser power output is measured in watts. The number of watts applied to a square centimeter (watts/cm^2) of tissue equals the power density. Power density can be increased by using more watts or, much more effectively, by reducing the surface area of the tissue irradiated. Spot size is a measure of the surface area on which laser light is concentrated. Since density varies as the inverse of the area, reducing the spot size increases dramatically the power density.[7] The thermal effect produced—be it no effect, gentle warming, coagulation, necrosis, vaporization, or cutting—is directly related to the power density.

Energy density is a measure of the total amount of irradiation applied to tissue, or power density $\times$ seconds (watt·seconds/cm^2 or joules/cm^2).

The spectral absorption characteristics, or laser light interaction with different tissues, varies with the wavelength emitted. For example, the argon laser emits visible light at a wavelength of 0.488 to 0.514 μm, which has a strong affinity for hemoglobin and melanin. This wavelength is useful in a variety of human dermatologic applications, including removal of tattoos and port wine stains and in ophthalmology for treatment of retinal bleeding.

The CO$_2$ laser emits laser light in the non-visible far infrared spectrum of light at a wavelength of 10.6 μm. This wavelength is strongly absorbed by tissue water, making the CO$_2$ laser an excellent, precise cutting tool but with only poor to fair coagulating capability. Unfortunately, at this wavelength there is no silica fiber transmission. Laser energy is delivered to tissue by a rigid hand piece connected to an articulating arm containing a complex series of mirrors. This makes only line-of-sight fire possible, limiting its usefulness in the horse's upper respiratory tract. While transendoscopic surgery with the CO$_2$ laser using flexible fiberoptics is not currently possible, manufacturers have been working for a number of years on a flexible wave guide delivery system. Commercial availability of such a system would make the CO$_2$ laser useful for equine upper respiratory surgery. Precise cartilage and mucosal cutting might be possible in a standing, awake patient on an outpatient basis.

Currently only the Nd:YAG laser energy at a wavelength of 1.06 μm is capable of being transmitted through a flexible optical quartz fiber. These fibers are either 1.8 (pediatric) or 2.2 (standard) mm OD and readily pass through the biopsy channel of all commercially available flexible fiberoptic and video endoscopes. YAG light is in the near infrared wavelength and, hence, is not visible. A visible helium neon laser aiming light is emitted from the fiber, facilitating accurate placement of the fiber tip. Since YAG light passes through water, it can be used in fluid-filled body cavities, such as the urinary bladder, and in the presence of hemorrhage.[7] The fiber tip protruding from the end of the endoscope is seen and laser energy is applied to tissue in either non-contact or contact fashion.

NON-CONTACT VERSUS CONTACT CONCEPTS

In non-contact applications, the fiber is held approximately 3 to 5 mm from the tissue and must not touch the tissue. In a non-contact system, if the fiber contacts blood or tissue, it must be withdrawn and subsequently recleaved or polished. YAG light is absorbed diffusely by all protein molecules and, when used non-contact, the laser light penetrates to a depth of approximately 3 to 5 mm. The YAG laser used for non-contact has excellent coagulating and tissue vaporization capabilities but is only a fair tissue cutter. Higher energy levels in the range of 40 to 100 watts are usually needed. Smoke plume production may necessitate use of a commercially available smoke evacuator. Substantial forward, lateral, and back scatter can create significant tissue effects that are not immediately apparent. The delayed thermal effects may result in subsequent tissue necrosis and sloughing. This characteristic is a problem where precision is essential but can be used to the surgeon's advantage for treating certain conditions, such as ethmoid hematomas or larger pharyngeal polyps for which a bulk heating effect may be desirable.

With the advent of contact laser tips (first developed by Surgical Laser Technologies in 1985)* contact delivery of YAG energy to tissue became possible. This delivery method overcomes many of the limitations of conventional non-contact medical laser systems. Energy loss to back scatter is less than 5% and the usual laser power output needed to achieve a given therapeutic effect is 75% to 90% lower than needed in a non-contact procedure.[7] Cutting, vaporization, and coagulation are possible with fewer than 25 watts of power.

Contact tips are made of a synthetic sapphire crystal, which has a melting point of 2,030 to 2,050°C. They are attached to a metal threaded universal connector, which screws onto the fiber tip. Coaxial tip cooling is achieved with either air or sterile fluid delivered through portals on either side of the probe. Probes come in different shapes, such as round, flat, chisel, conical, frosted, and laser scalpel. The probe configuration determines which tissue effect is produced. By simply withdrawing the fiber from the endoscope biopsy channel, a new or different type probe can be attached in seconds without having to withdraw the endoscope from the patient. Blood and tissue debris do not affect tip performance.

Endoscopic direct vision or video endoscopy viewed on a television monitor gives a two-dimensional picture, thereby making an accurate estimation of depth perception difficult. Differences in angle of inclination and irregularities in tissue contour also complicate

---

*Surgical Laser Technologies, One Great Valley Parkway, Suite 20, Malvern, PA 19355.

transendoscopic non-contact laser application. Contact tips reduce this problem by returning the surgeon's tactile sense.

Also, by reducing the spot size with a contact tip, high enough power densities can be achieved with YAG energy to provide good cutting capability with minimal damage to adjacent tissue. Smoke production and lateral heat transfer are substantially reduced compared to non-contact YAG techniques.

LASER TECHNIQUE IN EQUINE SURGERY

The goal of transendoscopic laser surgery is to reduce the morbidity and convalescence associated with conventional invasive procedures. Most procedures can be performed on an outpatient basis with the horse standing in stocks using short-acting xylazine sedation supplemented with topical anesthesia. A laryngotomy and the attendant postoperative care is eliminated. A sterile incision is produced, and hemorrhage is greatly reduced, particularly when operating on highly vascular tissue. Healing following laser surgery is rapid. In human patients, pain, swelling, and scarring are reportedly reduced compared with other techniques. Depending somewhat on the location and nature of the lesion, most horses are able to return to competitive work in 7 to 14 days. A few lesions, primarily because of their location, are best approached with the horse under general anesthesia.

The major disadvantage of laser surgery is equipment cost and the need for surgeon training. New lasers range from $60,000 to $100,000; however, used, reconditioned equipment is becoming more readily available as lasers are becoming more widely used. There are many reasonably priced, excellent instructional courses held throughout the country on a regular basis, which offer didactic and hands-on training leading to laser certification. Equipment expense alone is likely to restrict laser acquisition to university and large private equine surgical referral facilities that examine a high percentage of race horses.

Safety guidelines

Safety is an integral part of laser surgery.[4] Certifying courses are essential for both clinicians and nurses. Laser surgery is performed in a room where access can be controlled and windows must be covered to avoid inadvertent ocular exposure to potentially harmful laser energy. YAG laser energy passes through fluid and can be absorbed by the retina. Therefore, special warning signs are posted and protective glasses, designed to filter out the wavelength of light emitted by the particular laser in use, are worn by everyone in the room. Ocular danger to the horse is avoided by performing surgery transendoscopically within an enclosed body cavity with the image viewed on a television monitor. Protective filters attached to the endoscope eyepiece can be used if direct viewing is used, eliminating the need for protective glasses. For transendoscopic procedures viewed on a television monitor, glasses are not considered necessary. In our hospital, protective glasses are always worn because of the number of inexperienced people watching laser surgery.

Equipment

The SLT model CL-60 contact laser system★ generates up to 60 watts of power for non-contact use and is extremely stable at lower powers when used for contact surgery. This laser is completely enclosed and portable, has its own internal cooling system, and operates on standard 220 voltage. Laser operation is simplified by a microprocessor that projects easy-to-understand instructions onto a plasma screen at the top of the laser. The CL-60 is reliable, and maintenance has been reasonable to date.

A good quality 1 m flexible fiberoptic endoscope† with a good quality light source or, preferably, a 1 m laser-designated video endoscope‡ is necessary. On the last 125 upper respiratory cases I operated on with the YAG laser, I used a lightweight camera,§ designed primarily for arthroscopy, attached by an adapter to an Olympus fiberoptic endoscope (Fig. 8-1). While use of the camera reduces image clarity and brightness on the television monitor, it does facilitate endoscope positioning by the assistant. The video endoscopy light source we recently acquired provides a superior image when used with either the fiberoptic adapter or the video endoscope. This improves speed and accuracy in completing the procedure and reduces operator fatigue.

When in a laser-ready mode, care is taken that the probe and fiber are *continually* seen protruding through the endoscope tip to prevent inadvertent damage to the biopsy channel caused by firing the laser while the fiber was within the biopsy channel. When removing the fiber the laser is placed on standby.

Four additional pieces of equipment have proved extremely useful (Fig. 8-2): a broncho-esophagoscopic Universal grasping forceps, a steel guide tube, a snare, and a curved probe with a circular angled backstop.

A 600 mm length broncho-esophagoscopic Universal grasping

★See footnote on p. 87.

†Olympus Gastrointestinal Fiberscope, 9150 Rumsey Road, Suite A-4, Columbia, MD 21045

‡Welch Allyn, Video Division, State Street Road, Box 220, Skaneateles Falls, NY 13153-0220.

§Circon Corporation, 749 Ward Drive, Santa Barbara, CA 93111.

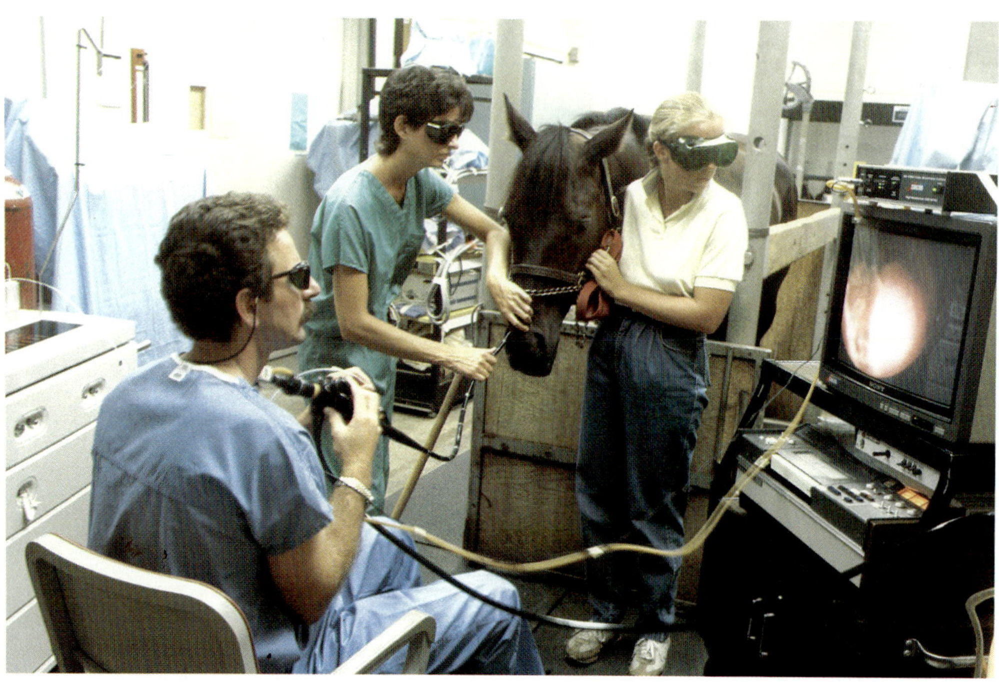

FIG. 8-1 YAG laser surgery room during routine correction of epiglottic entrapment. The laser is seen to the viewer's left and the television monitor to the viewer's right. Protective glasses are being worn and windows are covered for safety.

forceps* with 4 mm OD jaws can be used to retrieve large tissue fragments from the nasal passages and dorsal pharyngeal recess. When inserted into a custom-designed 56 cm long steel guide tube† (10 mm OD, 6 mm ID), the forceps allows access to all areas of the pharynx, larynx, and proximal trachea up to 60 cm from the nares. The forceps guide tube is inserted into the nasal passage opposite the endoscope and advanced into view. Next, the forceps are introduced into the guide tube and advanced until the jaws protrude from the guide tube end. While using the arthroscopic principle of triangulation, view the lesion and grasp it.[3] The forceps are removed and cleaned, leaving the guide tube in the nasal passage, eliminating the need for repeated passage of the tube.

The third instrument is a custom-designed snare made from a metal mare urinary catheter and a 2 m long piece of obstetric wire. Increasing the radius of curvature in the mid to distal third of the catheter makes this an ideal snare for a transoral approach to subepiglottic cysts. The obstetric wire is passed up the catheter and

---

*Universal broncho-esophagoscopic Grasping Forceps, 600 mm length, #8280.62, Richard Wolf Medical Instrument Corporation, 7046 Lindon Avenue, Rosemont, IL 60018.

†Guide Tube, custom-designed by Dr. Eric Tulleners, University of Pennsylvania, manufactured by Longwood Manufacturing Corporation, 816 E. Baltimore Pike, Kennett Square, PA 19348.

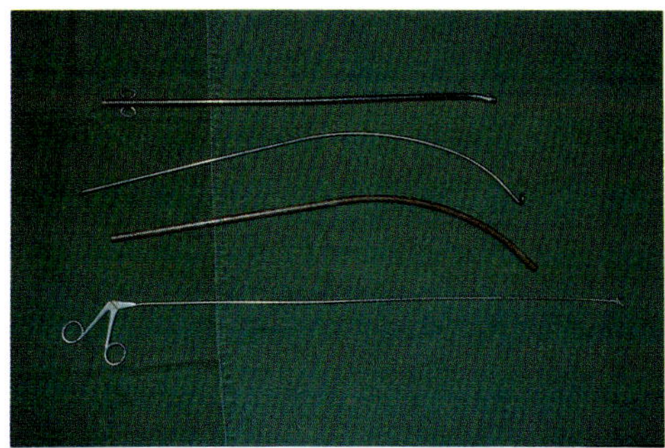

FIG. 8-2 Equipment recommended for equine laser upper respiratory tract surgery. From bottom to top: 600 mm Universal broncho-esophagoscopic grasping forceps, custom designed forceps guide tube, curved probe with circular angled backstop, and a custom designed snare.

through the end side portal. The wire is introduced back into the side portal and threaded retrograde until it exits the end, while maintaining a loop protruding from the side portal. Handles may be attached to the two wire ends protruding from the catheter. The wire loop and catheter are advanced into the mouth digitally with the horse under general anesthesia in lateral recumbency and the catheter tip is positioned ventral to the epiglottis. The loop is positioned around the remaining attachments of the subepiglottic cyst and the wire is tightened by an assistant. Final positioning is confirmed endoscopically with the endoscope introduced into the oropharynx through the mouth. The surgeon maintains positioning and stability of the snare intraorally while the assistant completes the cut. The snare and cyst are then removed from the mouth.

The fourth instrument is a curved probe with a circular angled back stop* which is introduced into the mouth and used to retract the soft palate.

Restraint

After performing a complete physical and endoscopic examination and radiography, if indicated, the horse is sedated with 0.4 mg/kg xylazine intravenously and restrained in stocks. The horse's head is suspended at a normal height in crossties. The lesion is visualized with the endoscope and an appropriate length of PE 240 tubing† is advanced through the biopsy channel until the tubing can be seen. The lesion is then sprayed with topical anesthetic‡ until anesthesia is achieved. Additional increments of 0.2 mg/kg xylazine are given

---

*Curved probe with a circular angled backstop, custom-designed by Dr. Eric Tulleners, University of Pennsylvania, manufactured by Longwood Manufacturing Corporation, 816 E. Baltimore Pike, Kennett Square, PA 19348.
†PE 240 tubing, Intramedic non-radiopaque polyethylene tubing. Clay Adams, Division of Becton Dickinson and Company, Parsippany, NJ 07054.
‡Cetacaine, topical anesthetic spray. Cetylite Industries Inc., 9051 River Road, Pennsauken, NJ 08110.

intravenously as needed to promote sedation and analgesia. In procedures lasting less than 30 minutes, usually one additional dose of xylazine is necessary. If the procedure takes longer than 30 minutes, respraying the lesion with topical anesthetic may be necessary. A twitch is infrequently used, and no other form of sedation or analgesia has been necessary. One assistant governs the endoscope positioning while another stands by on the opposite side of the horse to provide restraint if necessary (Fig. 8-1).

LASER SURGERY GUIDELINES BY ANATOMICAL LOCATION (TABLE 1)

Nasal septum/turbinates

Hemorrhage. On rare occasions, small erosive lesions on the nasal septum or turbinates cause recurrent mild hemorrhage. In humans, a flat contact probe is used transendoscopically for coagulation of bleeding gastric ulcers. A rosette is formed around the bleeding site by repeated applications of the round probe at 8 to 10 watts for 1 to 2 second intervals. This heats the tissues sufficiently to produce edema and protein coagulation causing hemostasis.[7] Once active bleeding subsides, if a discrete vessel is identified, the exposed end can be sealed directly. Vessels up to 3 mm in diameter can be safely sealed with this technique.[7]

Infection (bacterial or mycotic). The contact chisel probe is excellent for planing (shaving) and excising tissue in layers. At 12 to 15 watts it creates a clean, bloodless cut when advanced slowly with one flat surface against tissue. Necrotic tissue can be gently undermined and then removed with the grasping forceps. Photovaporization with higher powers used in the non-contact method might also be considered (Fig. 8-3).

Enlargement of the nasal maxillary opening. As an adjunct to maxillary sinus surgery, enlargement of the existing nasomaxillary opening is often desirable to provide drainage. The YAG laser can be used non-contact transendoscopically to photovaporize this tissue and create a larger opening.

Ethmoid turbinates

If given sufficient time and left untreated, most ethmoid hematomas expand into the frontal and/or maxillary sinuses, nasal passages, and even the pharynx. Except at their origination site from the ethmoid turbinates, they do not appear to be invasive or to have firm, discrete attachments to adjacent tissue. While their biologic activity varies considerably, ethmoid hematomas are usually slow-expanding, space-occupying lesions that may become debilitating to the horse if they become large enough to reduce nasal pharyngeal airflow and result in recurrent epistaxis.

TABLE 8-1 Transendoscopic upper respiratory YAG laser applications in horses

ANATOMICAL LOCATION/DISEASE	RECOMMENDED TREATMENT
Nasal septum/turbinate	
Recurrent mild hemorrhage—erosive lesion	Cauterize with a flat probe
Infection—bacterial, mycotic	Chisel probe debridement or photovaporize non-contact
Enlarged nasomaxillary opening	Photovaporize non-contact
Ethmoid turbinates	
Ethmoid hematoma	
Small (<5 cm diameter) initial or recurrent	Chisel probe excision and forceps retrieval or photovaporize non-contact
Large (>5 cm diameter +/− sinus involvement)	Base (stalk) excision★
Pharyngeal vault	
Solitary polyps	Chisel probe excision with forceps retrieval
Diffuse pharyngitis	Photovaporize non-contact
Cysts—dorsal, pharyngeal recess	Chisel probe excision and forceps retrieval
Guttural pouch	
Tympanites	Establish communication through the septum with a chisel probe
Epiglottis	
Dorsal abscess	Chisel probe incision and debridement
Epiglottic entrapment	Chisel probe division
Subepiglottic cyst†	Chisel probe excision and forceps retrieval
Arytenoid	
Chondroma—granulation tissue	Chisel probe excision and forceps retrieval
Laryngeal ventricle	
Ventriculectomy	Chisel probe excision or photovaporization non-contact
Dorsal larynx—trachea	
Granulation tissue	Chisel probe excision and forceps retrieval
Suture (laryngoplasty penetration)	Chisel probe excision and forceps retrieval
Injection granuloma	Chisel probe excision and forceps retrieval
Necrotic ulceration	Chisel probe debridement and biopsy instrument retrieval

★Requires general anesthesia, sinusotomy flap, and a 0.6 to 1.2 mm laser scalpel.
†Requires general anesthesia and an oral approach, forceps, and a snare.

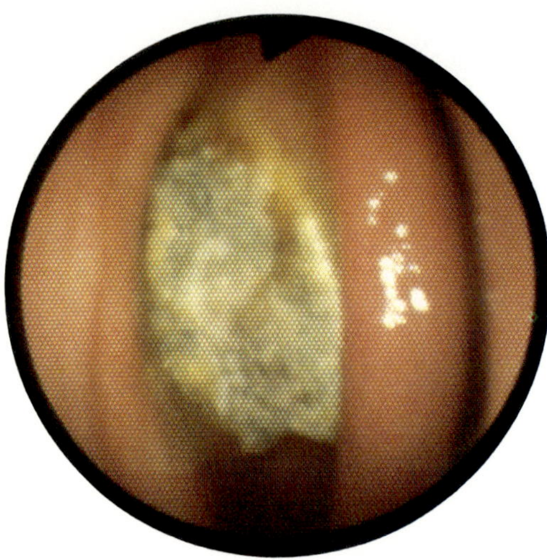

FIG. 8-3   Mycotic plaque in the right nasal passage amenable to transendoscopic laser debridement.

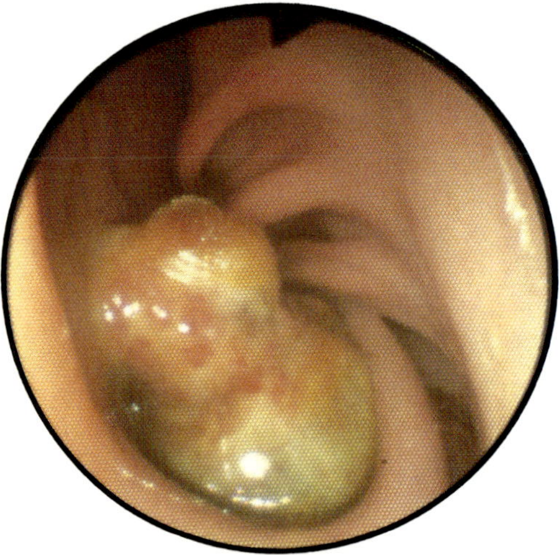

FIG. 8-4   Small ethmoid hematoma in the medial aspect of the left ethmoid recess. This lesion was treated successfully with a chisel probe and forceps removal.

Most ethmoid hematomas are visible with the endoscope from an end-on view within the ethmoid turbinates positioned dorsally approximately 30 cm from the nares in adult horses. One horse was brought in with intermittent, scant, unilateral nasal epistaxis and had blood emanating from the nasomaxillary opening. No abnormality of the ethmoid turbinates was observed during endoscopic examination. Maxillary sinus radiography revealed a large soft tissue density mass in the affected sinus. An exploratory maxillary sinusotomy revealed a large ethmoid hematoma which had grown laterally from the ethmoid turbinate through the frontal maxillary opening. Radiographs are recommended to determine the full extent of the lesion.

Much of the hemorrhage historically associated with excision of ethmoid hematomas through traditional flap techniques may be associated with trauma to highly vascular adjacent tissues, such as the turbinates and nasal septum. Small lesions (less than 5 cm in diameter) that do not invade the sinuses may be safely approached transendoscopically, with the horse standing, using either the non-contact or contact technique (Fig. 8-4). When using the non-contact method the mass is photovaporized. Coagulated and necrotic tissue can be removed with forceps, and very small lesions can be treated in one procedure. Larger lesions may require sequential debridement on an every-other-day or twice-weekly schedule if light bleeding obscures the view. Using a round or chisel probe and the contact technique, the hematoma is coagulated and divided into pieces. A forceps is then used to retrieve larger fragments. In either technique, the hematoma, ideally, should be ablated down to the stalk to reduce recurrence. Access to and visualization of these smaller hematomas are superior to that obtained by conventional bone flap techniques, and hemostasis is excellent.[2] Horses tolerate this procedure without signs of discomfort, and use of general anesthesia is avoided. Small recurrent or incompletely ablated lesions may be treated periodically to avoid major surgery.

Large hematomas that have invaded the sinuses may be treated non-contact with sequential photovaporization although progress is slow. These extensive lesions may be best approached (with the horse under general anesthesia) through a dorsally-based curvilinear flap approximately 3 cm wide × 6 cm long, made medial to the eye beginning just below the supraorbital foramen. The hematoma is carefully separated digitally from adjacent mucosa. By using a 0.6 mm hand-held laser scalpel and 15 watts of power, the stalk is transected at the base. The hematoma is then teased out of the flap opening (Fig. 8-5).

Hemorrhage is usually greatly reduced with this technique, unless adjacent tissue is inadvertently disturbed. Transfusions have not been necessary. The nasal passage and sinus are packed routinely,

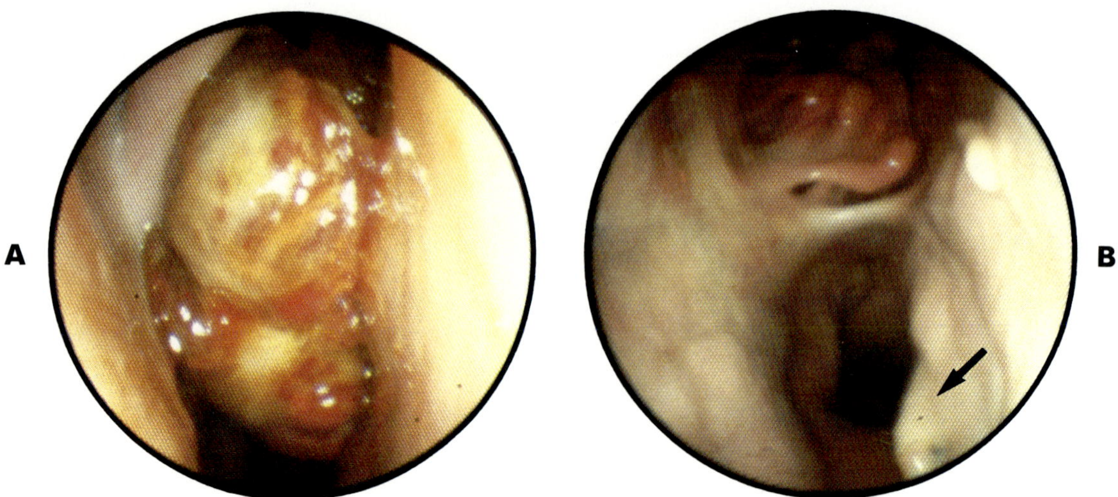

FIG. 8-5   **A**, Large, right-sided ethmoid hematoma with maxillary sinus involvement. **B**, Right nasal passage looking up into the ethmoid recess one year after laser scalpel excision of the ethmoid hematoma stalk through a bone flap. Note the nasal septum irregularity on the viewer's right caused by chronic pressure exerted by the hematoma *(arrow)*. **C**, Close-up of remaining right ethmoturbinate one year after laser scalpel excision of an ethmoid hematoma. Arrow denotes stalk excision site.

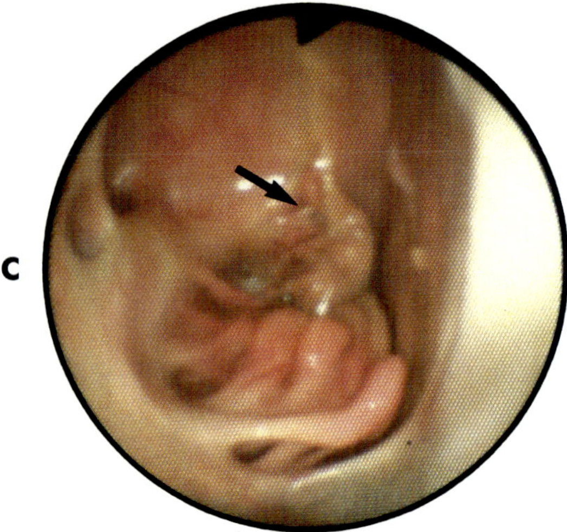

with the packing material made to exit from the nares for subsequent retrieval. Flap closure and postoperative care are routine. For unilateral lesions a tracheotomy has not been necessary. Packing is usually removed in 48 hours. If the flap is healing routinely and endoscopic examination is unremarkable, the horse can return to work in 30 days. Usually at 30 days the ethmoid recess is covered with a healthy appearing mucous membrane.

Pharyngeal vault

Polyps. Occasionally, large, solitary polyps containing lymphoid tissue persist as the horse matures. If clinically indicated, they can be photovaporized via the non-contact modality or, preferably, excised with a chisel probe and 15 watts of power (Fig. 8-6). The excised masses are removed with the grasping forceps within the guide tube. Phenylbutazone is given once postoperatively, and no other postoperative care is necessary. Training is usually resumed in one week following endoscopic reexamination.

Diffuse pharyngitis. Pharyngitis can be treated via the non-contact modality with 40 to 60 watts applied in a sweeping pattern to affected areas of the pharynx until the tissue blanches and grays slightly. Postoperatively, phenylbutazone (2 mg/kg orally twice daily for 7 days) is given to reduce inflammation. The horse is confined for 30 days, and exercise is resumed after re-examination.

Dorsal pharyngeal cysts. These large, soft, grape clusterlike masses are rare but occasionally seen emanating from the dorsal pharyngeal recess (Fig. 8-7, *A*). By placing traction on the protruding mass with the straight grasping forceps without the guide tube, the base is exposed and incised with the chisel probe using 15 watts of power in 3 second pulses. Hemorrhage is minimal, and the mass can be removed through the nasal passages for histologic examination. (Fig. 8-7, *B*). Postoperative care consists of 2 mg/kg phenylbutazone given orally twice daily for 6 days and 1 week of stall confinement. Residual tissue retracts into the recess and heals by epithelialization and contraction.

Guttural pouch

Tympanites. Unilateral tympanites seen in foals usually respond to creation of a permanent stoma in the vertical mucosal septum separating the two guttural pouches. Traditionally this fenestration has been created with scissors introduced into the guttural pouch through a Viborgs triangle approach with the foal under general anesthesia. I have not done this procedure with the laser, but it seems feasible transendoscopically with the animal standing and sedated or under general anesthesia. The pediatric endoscope is easier to introduce into a foal's guttural pouch. A 1.8 mm pediatric fiber used non-contact or preferably with a round or chisel probe

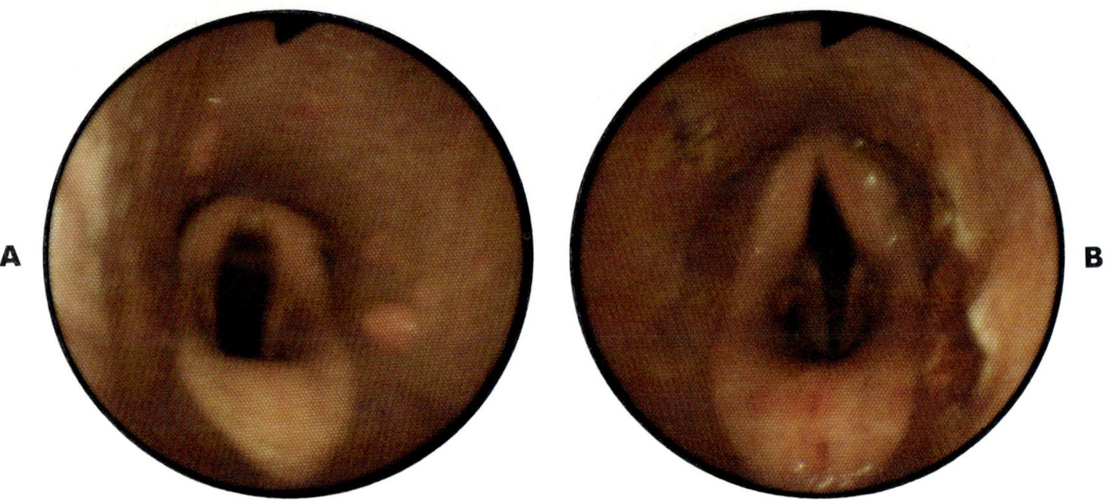

FIG. 8-6 **A**, Pharyngeal lymphoid polyps in a 3-year-old Thoroughbred racehorse. **B**, Immediate post–chisel probe excision appearance.

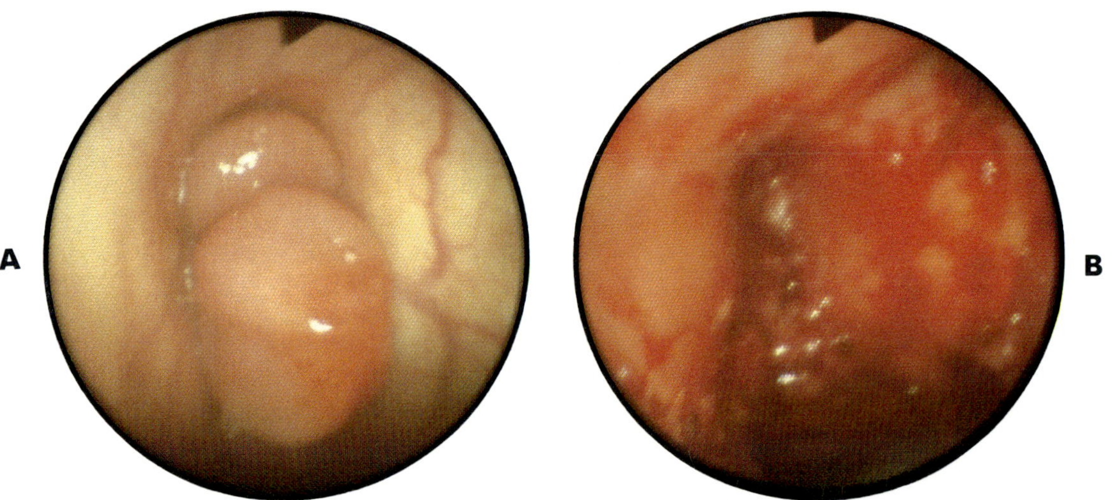

FIG. 8-7 **A**, Large dorsal pharyngeal recess cysts in a 3-year-old Thoroughbred racehorse. **B**, immediate post–chisel probe excision appearance.

would then be used to create the opening between the two guttural pouches in the same location where scissors would have been used.

Epiglottis

Dorsal epiglottic abscess.   Rarely, a submucosal abscess develops between the tightly adherent dorsal mucous membrane and the epiglottic cartilage (Fig. 8-8, *A*). This lesion is painful to the horse, causing intermittent dorsal displacement of the soft palate and sometimes coughing during deglutition. The abscess can be incised on its cranial aspect either vertically or transversely with a chisel probe (15 watts of power and 3 second pulses) to allow for drainage. Inspissated material can be removed and the interior debrided with the grasping forceps within the tube guide (Fig. 8-8, *B*). Dorsal epiglottic granulomas may be treated in a similar manner (Fig. 8-8, *C*).

Epiglottic entrapment.   Epiglottic entrapment by the aryepiglottic folds is a very commonly diagnosed cause of decreased exercise tolerance and respiratory noise, particularly in racehorses (Fig. 8-9, *A*). This lesion is ideal for YAG laser correction because a single midline division of the entrapping membranes has been shown to be effective in resolving the problem permanently in approximately 95% of cases.[9] Midline division may be preferable to traditional surgical techniques in which tissue is excised because of the number of horses with epiglottic entrapment that are concurrently affected by epiglottic hypoplasia. By preserving this normally ventrally located loose mucous membrane, bulk is not eliminated and scarring may be decreased, reducing the incidence of subsequent dorsal displacement of the soft palate.[9]

The chisel probe is oriented vertically and 15 watts of power and 3-second pulses are used. A cut is made precisely on midline starting at the epiglottic tip and gently sliding caudal toward the base. The incision is gradually deepened, and as the membranes begin to spread they change from a tangential to a more vertical orientation relative to the horizontal epiglottic axis. At this point the epiglottic tip can be identified as a white, triangular structure shining translucently through a thin, overlying membrane. The remaining deep mucosal reflection of the aryepiglottic fold tissue is carefully divided from the base toward the tip. Once the cut is very close to the epiglottic cartilage tip, swallowing is induced and the entrapping membranes should retract into their normal ventral epiglottic position. The now transverse or oval-to-circular mucosal defect can often be seen by maneuvering the endoscope tip underneath the epiglottis. If, after watching multiple swallowing movements, there is no tendency to re-entrap, the procedure is terminated (Fig. 8-9, *B*). Occasionally, a narrow, border-like appearance is seen after swallowing, and a small amount of additional work must be performed

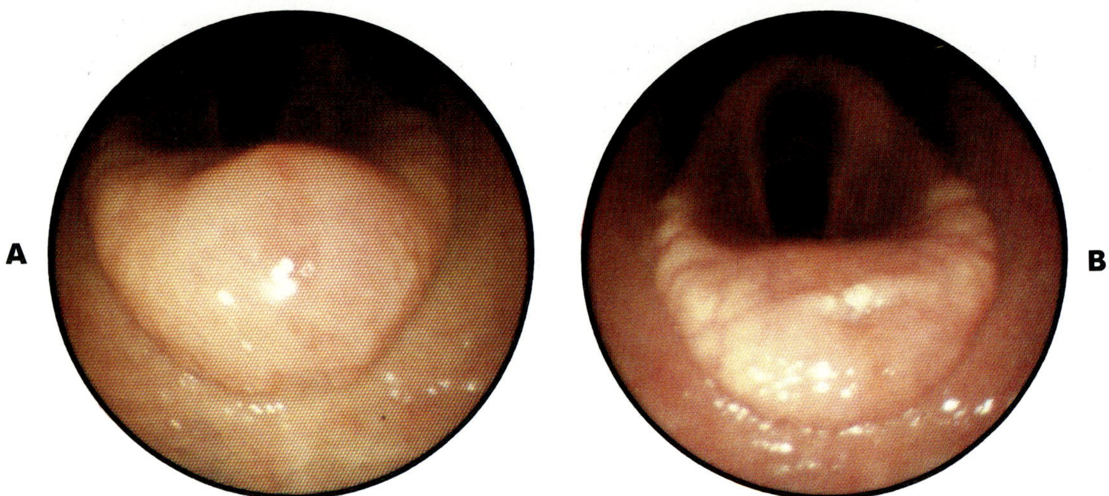

FIG. 8-8 **A**, Dorsal epiglottic abscess in a 4-year-old Thoroughbred racehorse. The abscess was incised vertically with a chisel probe. **B**, Ten days post-drainage debridement. The mucous membrane is flat and well healed with only a small residual scar. **C**, Dorsal epiglottic granuloma amenable to laser excision with a chisel probe. (Photograph courtesy of Dr. Charles W. Raker, Professor Emeritus of Surgery, University of Pennsylvania.)

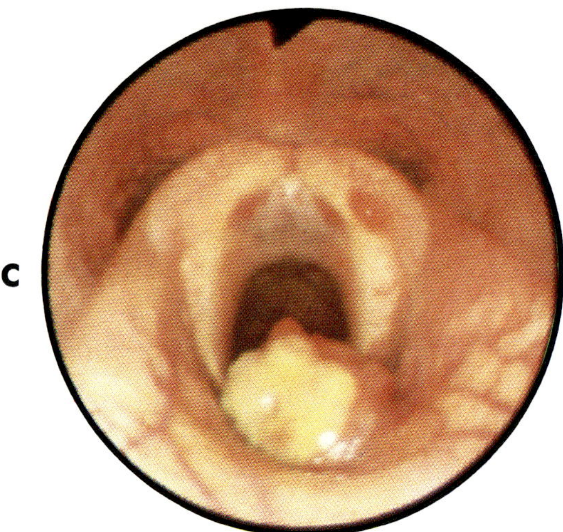

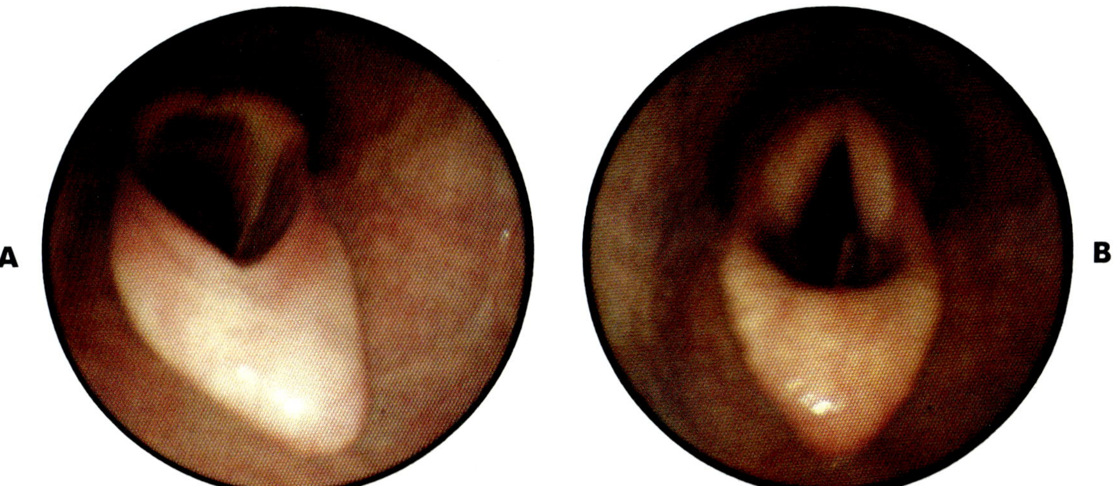

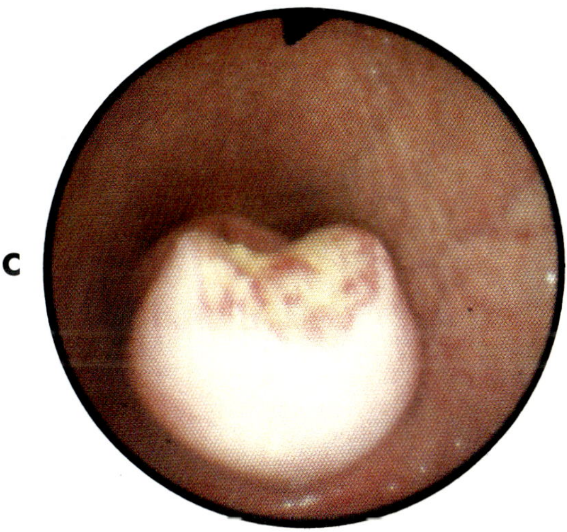

FIG. 8-9 **A**, A typical thick epiglottic entrapment in a Thoroughbred racehorse. **B**, Immediate postoperative appearance after midline division of the entrapping aryepiglottic fold membrane with a chisel probe. **C**, Extremely thick, severely ulcerated chronic epiglottic entrapment. The glottis and normal triangular epiglottic contour is obscured by the entrapping membranes. This horse was successfully treated via laryngotomy by resection of the central third of the aryepiglottic fold membranes.

adjacent to the tip. Large edematous pillars of mucous membrane are often seen laterally but are not of concern because they resolve with anti–inflammatory therapy in 7 to 14 days.

A complete, permanent, satisfactory correction is most difficult to achieve in horses that are severely hypoplastic; they lack sufficient epiglottic rigidity to maintain the aryepiglottic fold membranes in a normal ventral position.

Approximately 5% of horses are brought in with extremely thick, chronic entrapments that badly deform the epiglottic contour, primarily resulting from epiglottic malformation and/or hypoplasia (Fig. 8-9 *C*). If a satisfactory standing correction cannot be achieved, the only recourse is to perform a central third aryepiglottic fold resection via a laryngotomy incision with the horse under general anesthesia.[1] Rarely, a horse presents with severe hypoplasia, epiglottic entrapment, and almost persistent dorsal displacement of the soft palate. Standing correction of the epiglottic entrapment is usually not possible because of persistent dorsal displacement of the soft palate. If in spite of the poor prognosis rendered for usefulness during fast exercise the owners request surgery, a central one third of the aryepiglottic fold resection and possibly a concomitant soft palate resection are done through a laryngotomy.

After routine laser correction of epiglottic entrapment, the horse is confined for one week. Phenylbutazone (2 mg/kg given orally twice daily for 6 days) is given after one intravenous injection of 5 mg/kg, immediately after surgery. Fifteen ml of a pharyngeal spray* is administered by the owner or trainer twice daily for one week through a #10 French catheter passed into the pharynx through the nasal passage. If, on repeated endoscopic examination, in one week the dorsal epiglottic surface is visible and free of entrapping membranes, the horse may be returned to work if desired. Usually there is some mild to moderate residual inflammation ventrally that resolves in an additional 1 to 2 weeks but does not generally prevent the horse from returning to exercise.

Subepiglottic cyst. All subepiglottic cysts in adults can be excised without a laryngotomy (Fig. 8-10 *A*). An attempt at non-contact photovaporization of smaller cysts may be done transendoscopically with the horse standing, but usually the deflated cyst seals over, and because the secretory lining was not removed, the cyst refills within days. In the standing horse, the cyst, once deflated, is almost impossible to reach, and in most horses manipulation of the subepiglottic area induces a strong swallow reflex. For those reasons, subepiglottic cysts are approached orally and transendoscopically with the horse under general anesthesia and in lateral recumbency. The soft palate is dorsally displaced digitally, and inhalation

---

*Pharyngeal spray, 750 ml furacin, 250 ml DMSO, 1000 ml glycerin, 2000 mg prednisolone.

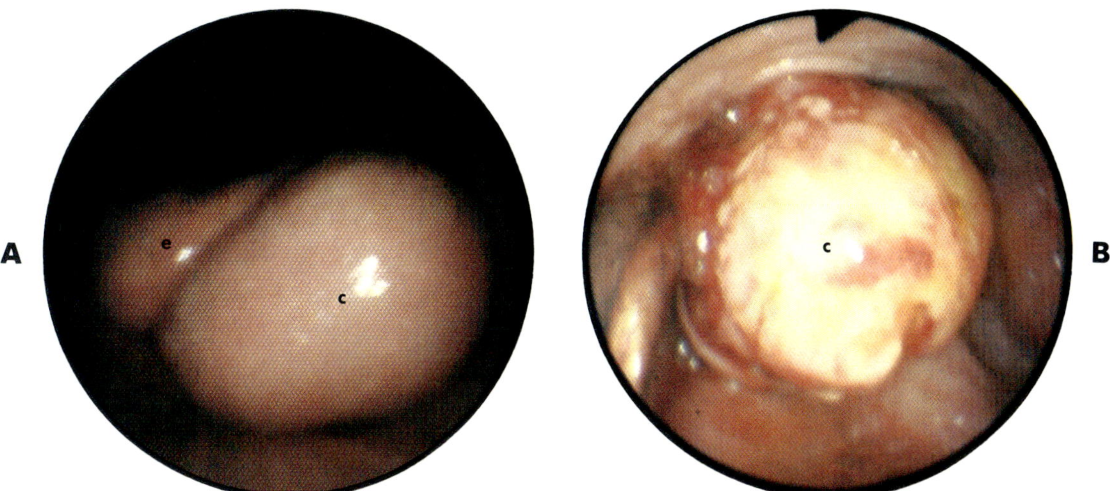

FIG. 8-10   **A**, Large subepiglottic cyst *(c)* to the viewer's right of the epiglottis*(e)* **B**, Intraoral view of the subepiglottic cyst with a snare in place to the viewer's left of the cyst. **C**, Appearance of epiglottis immediately after cyst excision.

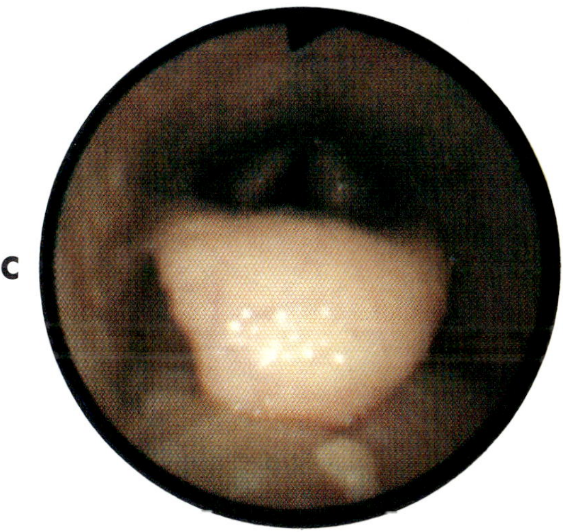

anesthesia is delivered through a nasal tracheal tube. Traction can be placed on the cyst with the grasping forceps within the guide tube. The chisel probe is used with 15 watts of power and 3-second pulses to incise the mucous membrane at the cyst stalk. If any residual tissue remains that cannot be accessed with the laser fiber, it is transected with the snare as previously described (Fig. 8-10, *B*). Hemorrhage is usually minimal (Fig. 8-10, *C*). Horses can return to work after one week of confinement and routine anti-inflammatory therapy.

Arytenoid chondroma

Partial arytenoidectomies have been performed using a CO_2 laser through a laryngotomy incision with the horse under general anesthesia.[5] When the CO_2 wave guide delivery system becomes commercially available, transendoscopic, standing, partial arytenoidectomy without mucosal closure may be possible and even preferable to conventional surgical excision. To date, a precise method of partial arytenoidectomy performed transendoscopically with a YAG laser, which yields reproducible results, has not been perfected.

Arytenoid chondropathy and failed laryngoplasty following treatment of laryngeal hemiplegia are the two most important reasons for performing an arytenoidectomy in a horse.[10] Occasionally, large granulation tissue masses project from the surface of the arytenoid cartilage, particularly on the medial side of the corniculate cartilage just above the vocal cord (Fig. 8-11 *A*). In the absence of significant underlying cartilage thickening and alteration in normal range of motion necessitating conventional partial arytenoidectomy, these projections can be managed by transendoscopic excision with the laser. The chisel probe, with 15 watts of power and 3-second pulses, is used to undermine the granulation tissue base circumferentially. Once the vascular supply has been dealt with and the mass is hanging loosely attached, it can be removed with the grasping forceps within the tube guide. This leaves a crater defect with smooth mucosal margins that heals by epithelialization and contraction (Fig. 8-11 *B*). This technique does not prevent or reverse any underlying, ongoing cartilage pathology. However, it may palliatively return a performance horse to usefulness for a period of time before a major, definitive arytenoidectomy procedure is necessary. In broodmares and stallions, it may serve as a definitive procedure, eliminating the need for general anesthesia and surgery.

Ventriculectomy

A ventriculectomy can be done alone or as an adjunct to laryngoplasty technique with the horse standing or under general anesthe-

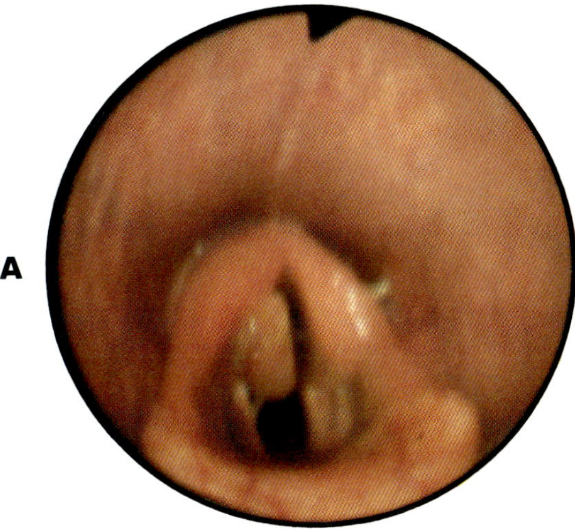

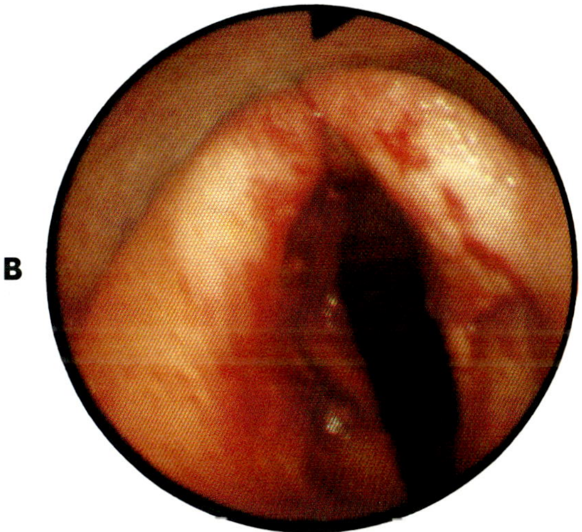

FIG. 8-11 **A**, Large granulation tissue mass protruding from the medial aspect of the corniculate process of the right arytenoid, just above the vocal cord. **B**, Appearance of corniculate process immediately after chisel probe excision of granulation tissue. Most of the hemorrhage resulted from use of large grasping forceps.

sia. In an experimental study, six horses each had one laryngeal ventricle photovaporized non-contact while under general (IV) anesthesia.[6] After the operation, all horses returned to eating without any problems. The horses were given phenylbutazone twice daily for 3 to 5 days, and no problems were noted. Endoscopic examination revealed almost complete sealing of the ventricles by day 42.[6] With the horse standing, ventriculectomy using the non-contact method has been successfully performed on clinical cases.[8] The contact technique using a chisel probe might also be possible.

Dorsal larynx and trachea

Laryngeal granulation tissue and exposed suture material. Occasionally, granulation tissue and exposed, non-absorbable suture material result from laryngoplasty placement with inadvertent mucosal penetration (Fig. 8-12, *A*). The chisel probe, with 15 watts of power and 3-second pulses, is used to undermine the granulation tissue. Granulation tissue and exposed suture material are removed with the grasping forceps within the tube guide (Fig. 8-12, *B*). Altering the head position will facilitate positioning of the forceps jaws into this hard to reach area.

Tracheal abscess. Necrotic tissue can be undermined and ulcers debrided effectively with the flat edge of the chisel probe, using 15 watts of power and 3-second pulses (Fig. 8-13, *A*). Tissue less than 60 cm from the nares can be removed with the large grasping forceps within the tube guide. Loose tissue in deeper than 60 cm that has been well-freed up can be grasped and removed with the biopsy forceps passed through the biopsy channel by slowly withdrawing the entire endoscope (Fig. 8-13, *B*).

Tracheal granulation tissue and injection granulomas can also be undermined and removed as described for tracheal abscesses (Fig. 8-14).

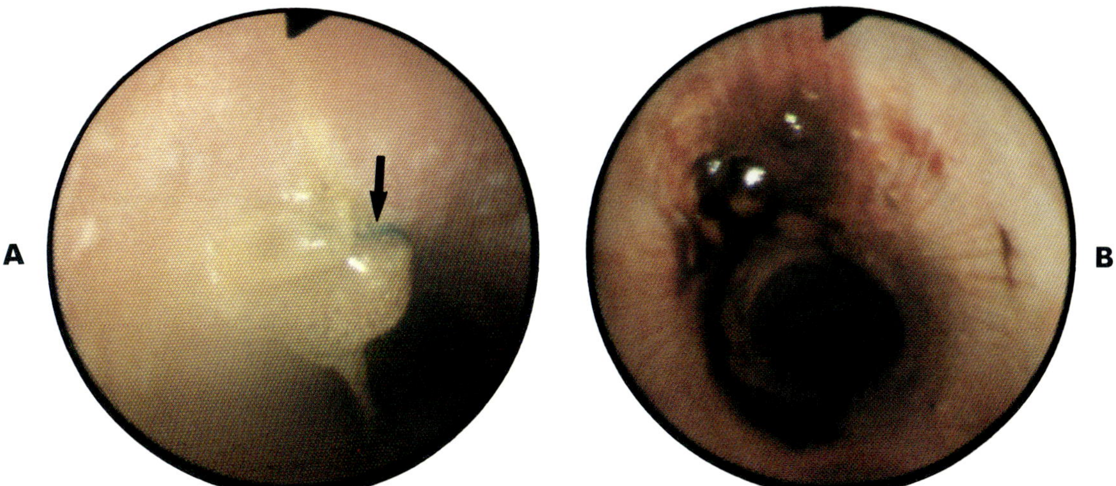

FIG. 8-12 **A**, Granulation tissue and exposed Mersilene suture material *(arrow)* in the dorsal right cricoid area following mucosal suture penetration during attempted laryngoplasty. **B**, Appearance immediately after chisel probe granulation tissue debridement and forceps–aided suture removal.

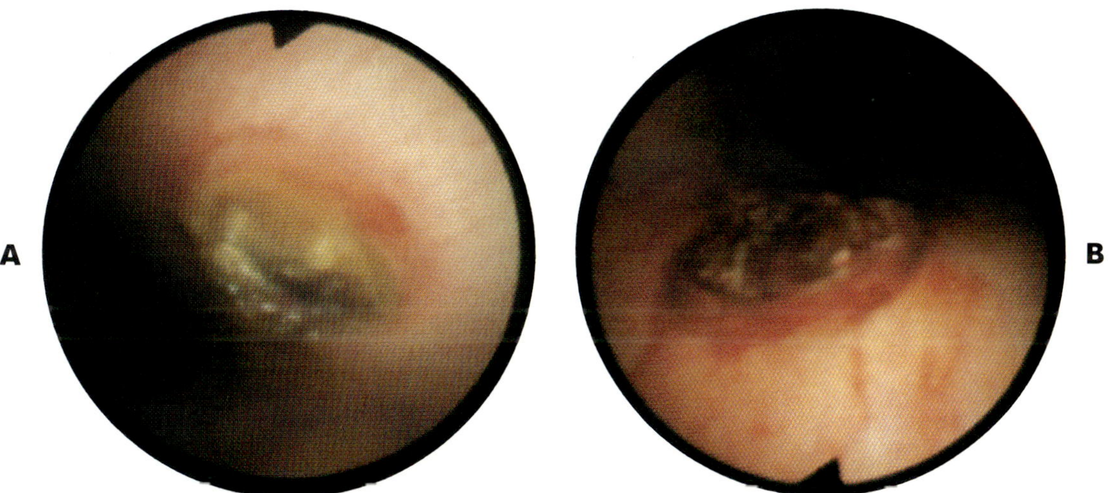

FIG. 8-13 **A**, Necrotic, non–healing, dorsal cervical tracheal ulcer 60 cm from the nares. **B**, Appearance immediately after chisel probe debridement. This defect was endoscopically healed in two weeks.

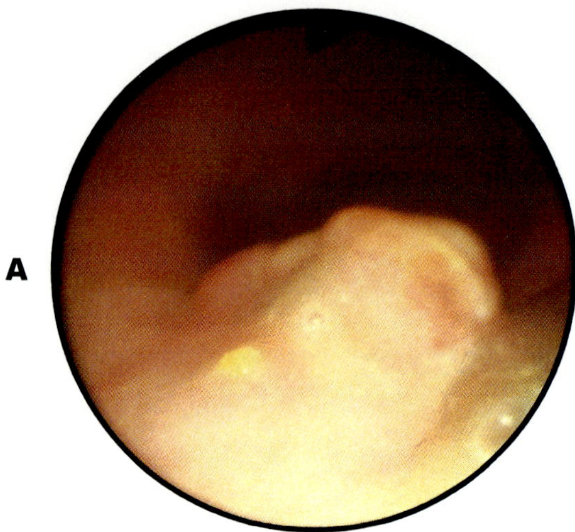

FIG. 8-14 **A**, Ventral cervical tracheal granuloma (15 mm in height by 6 cm long by 5 cm wide) in 60 to 70 cm from the nares. **B**, Appearance immediately after chisel probe and forceps excision.

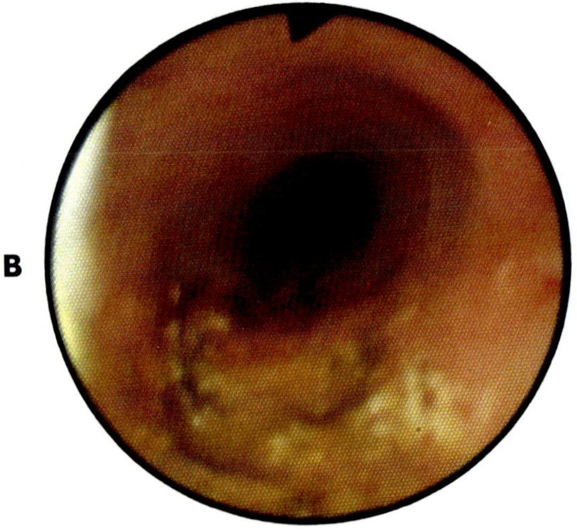

REFERENCES

1. Jann HW and Cook RW: Transendoscopic electrosurgery for epiglottic entrapment in the horse, J Am Vet Med Assoc 187(5):484, 1985.
2. Lloyd KC and Meagher DM: Nd:YAG laser treatment of ethmoid hematomas, Proc 125th Annual Convention, Am Vet Med Assoc, Portland, Ore., July, 1988.
3. McIlwraith WC: Diagnostic and surgical arthroscopy in the horse Edwardsville, Kansas, 1984 Vet Med Publishing Co.
4. Mohr RM et al: Safety considerations and safety protocol for laser surgery. Surg Clin North Am 64(5):851, Philadelphia, 1984.
5. Montgomery T: Personal communication. February, 1987, Louisville, KY.
6. Shires GM, Adair HS, and Patton CS: The use of the Nd:YAG laser for removal of the laryngeal ventricles in the equine: a pilot study, Proceedings 125th Annual Convention, Am Vet Med Assoc, Portland, Ore., July, 1988.
7. Surgical Laser Technologies: Contact laser surgery in endoscopy: an introduction, Monograph by SLT, Inc., 1 Great Valley Parkway, Malvern, Pa, 1985, pp. 1-16.
8. Tate, L: Personal communication. November, 1987, Raleigh, North Carolina.
9. Tulleners EP: Transendoscopic contact YAG laser correction of aryepiglottic fold entrapment in the standing horse: 24 cases, Vet Surg 17, 1988.
10. Tulleners EP, Harrison IW, and Raker CW: Management of arytenoid chondropathy and failed laryngoplasty in horses: 75 cases (1979-1985), J Am Vet Med Assoc 192(5):670, 1988.

Chapter 9

ESOPHAGUS

JOHN A. STICK

Esophagoscopy is an ancillary aid in the diagnosis of diseases of the equine esophagus. It should be performed when physical and radiographic examinations are not diagnostic; esophagoscopy may better define the severity and extent of lesions found on radiographic examination. In this chapter, other diagnostic and therapeutic considerations of esophageal disease in the horse have been largely omitted, and equine esophagoscopy, as it relates to diagnosis, is emphasized.

EXAMINATION OF THE ESOPHAGUS
Restraint

In most instances, endoscopic examination may be performed with the animal standing and physically restrained. The administration of xylazine (0.5 mg/kg of body weight) will greatly facilitate the examination by reducing the swallowing reflex and should be used when a physical obstruction or other painful condition is suspected. However, when lumen diameter or esophageal motility is being assessed (e.g., when megaesophagus is suspected) the use of chemical restraint should be avoided so that it will not interfere with interpretation of the examination.

Special equipment

If the endoscope is 150 cm or longer, the entire esophagus may be examined, and esophageal lesions in the thorax of the adult horse undetected on radiographic examination may be diagnosed. A flexible endoscope that allows irrigation and insufflation is necessary to provide good observation of mucosal disease and changes in luminal size.

Technique

Unless there is reason to suspect esophageal rupture, diagnostic observations are best made by starting with the endoscope fully inserted and the esophageal lumen insufflated. Then, the endoscope tip should be slowly withdrawn cranially (toward the head). After each swallow, the endoscope should be irrigated and the esophagus dilated before further withdrawal. Several passes should be made over any area of suspected disease.

NORMAL ENDOSCOPIC ANATOMY

Normal longitudinal mucosal folds of the esophagus are seen when the endoscope tip is moved cranially and the esophagus is in the relaxed position (Fig. 9-1). Insufflation flattens these folds and permits observation of luminal size (Fig. 9-2). An inability to insufflate the esophagus and flatten the longitudinal mucosal folds usually indicates a disease process. This will be noted cranial and caudal to a stricture. Transverse folds can be iatrogenically produced by moving the endoscope tip caudally (toward the stomach) (Fig. 9-3). When the cervical esophagus is insufflated, the outline of the trachea can often be seen through the esophageal wall. Swallowing produces changes in the lumen that give the appearance of diverticula (Fig. 9-4) or strictures (Fig. 9-5) to the untrained observer. The mucosa should appear white to light pink; reddened colorations are signs of mucosal disease.

The cranial aspect of the cervical esophageal sphincter is difficult to examine because repeated stimulation of the swallow reflex and the larynx directs the endoscope tip dorsally. Radiographic assessment of this area may be more diagnostic. Additionally, the longitudinal mucosal folds found along the rest of the esophagus are absent in this area (Fig. 9-6).

Frequently, the endoscopic appearance of an esophageal obstruction is obscured by saliva mixed with ingesta that collects cranial to it. This fluid should be removed by suction through a nasogastric tube, and the endoscope should be immediately reinserted to observe the obstruction.

ESOPHAGEAL ABNORMALITIES

Clinical manifestations of esophageal diseases in the horse usually result in luminal obstruction and, therefore, are similar regardless of

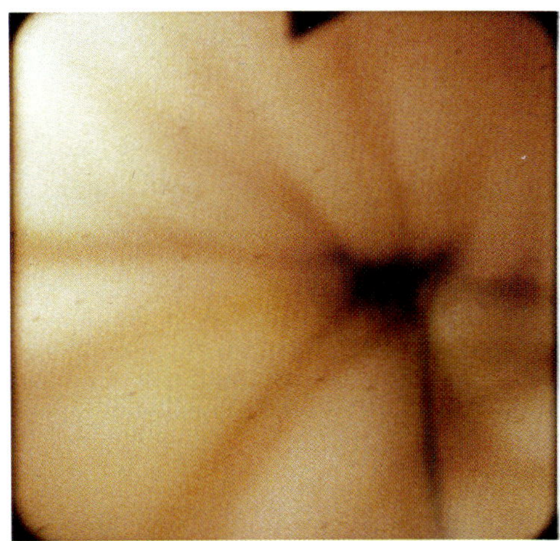

FIG. 9-1 Normal longitudinal mucosal folds are seen when the endoscope is fully inserted and then slowly withdrawn toward the patient's head without using insufflation.

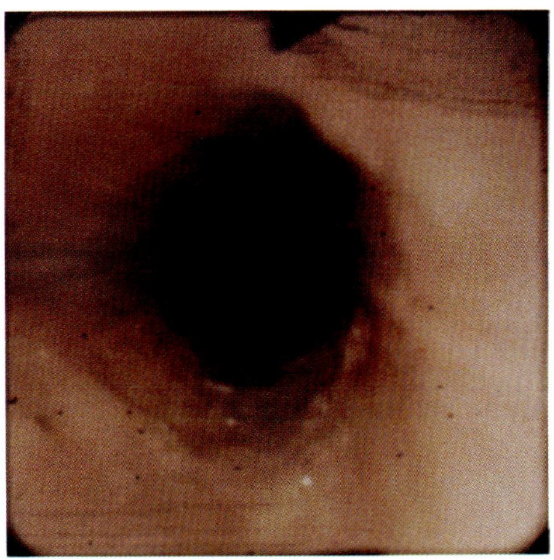

FIG. 9-2 Normal luminal size is observed when the esophagus is insufflated with air through the endoscope. This manipulation flattens the normal longitudinal mucosal folds.

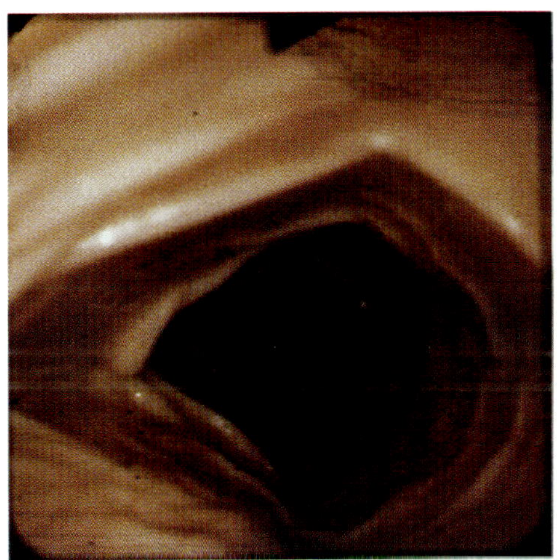

FIG. 9-3 Transverse folds can be iatrogenically produced by inserting the endoscope without insufflation.

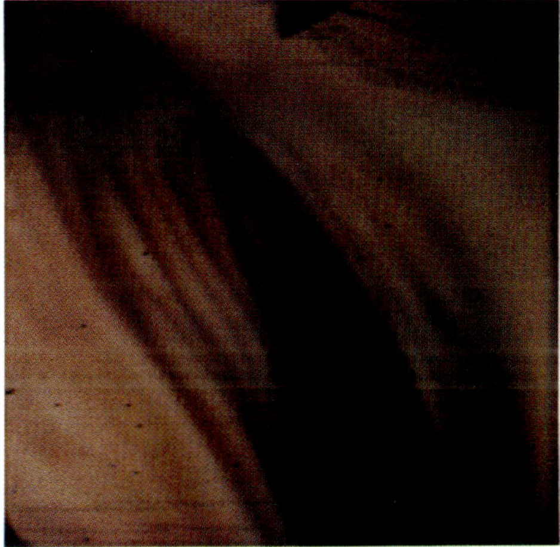

FIG. 9-4 Appearance of a false diverticulum in a normal esophagus after a swallow. Reinsufflation and examination of this area will produce a normal appearing lumen.

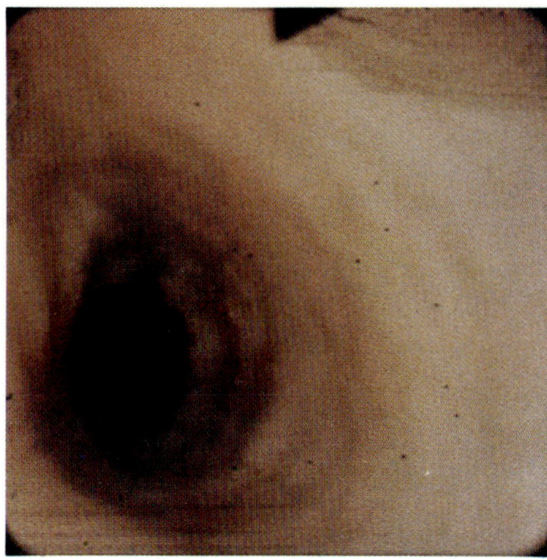

FIG. 9-5   Appearance of a false stricture in a normal esophagus after a swallow. The incidence of swallowing can be reduced by sedation with xylazine.

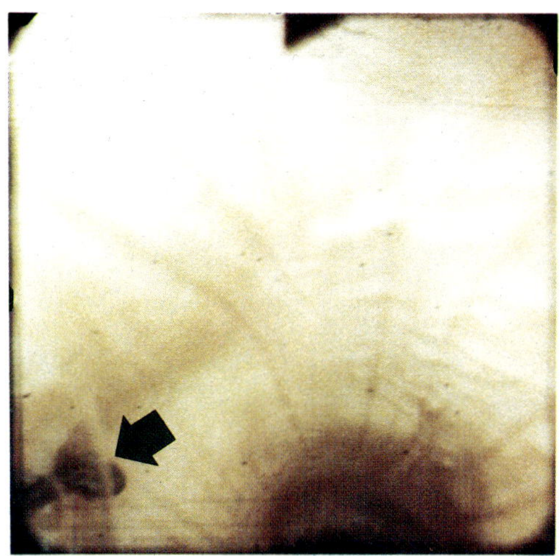

FIG. 9-6   Cranial aspect of the cervical esophagus just dorsal to the larynx is difficult to examine because the endoscope is held against the dorsal wall of the esophagus. Note the absence of longitudinal mucosal folds in this region and the eye of a fish hook *(arrow)* lodged in the cranial esophageal sphincter.

etiology. The manifestations of "choke" in the horse include: ptyalism; dysphagia; coughing; and regurgitation of food, water, and saliva from the mouth and nostrils. Attempts at ingestion are often followed by odynophagia (painful swallowing), repeated extension of the head and neck, and other signs of distress or agitation. The time interval from swallowing until these signs are shown by the patient will depend on the location of the lesion within the esophagus. With obstruction of the lower esophagus, odynophagia and retching may occur 10 to 12 seconds after swallowing. But when an upper esophageal obstruction is present, signs may be immediate.

Intermittent signs of choke followed by periods of relief may indicate a disease other than simple feed impaction, and further diagnostic procedures are warranted. Anorexia, electrolyte imbalances, and dehydration accompany cases of long duration. Aspiration pneumonia frequently follows esophageal obstruction, and signs may be present as early as one day after the onset of choke. Table 9-1 lists specific clinical signs that may be exhibited by a patient with a given esophageal abnormality.

TABLE 9-1 Esophageal abnormalities

CONDITION	CLINICAL SIGNS
Diverticulum (Figs. 9-7 and 9-8)	Intermittent signs of obstruction or enlargement of the neck in the area of the diverticulum
Foreign body (Fig. 9-6)	Hard, painful enlargement on the neck if sharp, foreign body has penetrated the lumen
Fistula (Fig. 9-9)	Salivary loss; food or water observed from fistula, especially when drinking
Megaesophagus (Fig. 9-10)	Signs of choke either at birth or when solid food is introduced
Impaction (Fig. 9-11)	Odynophagia is the most common sign.
Rupture (Fig. 9-12)	Phlegmon of the cervical region; fever; depression; shock
Stricture (Figs. 9-14 and 9-15)	Recurrence of choke
Ulceration (Figs. 9-13, 9-16 and 9-17)	Grinding of teeth in foals (associated with gastric ulceration); ptyalism

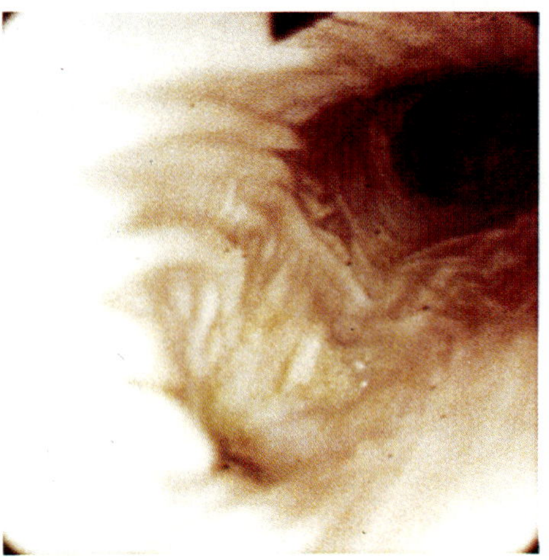

FIG. 9-7 A traction diverticulum has a wide neck that permits easy visualization into the sac and usually does not result in clinical signs of esophageal obstruction.

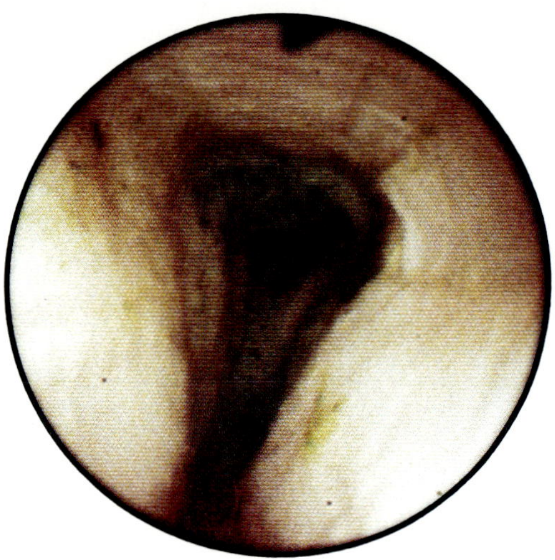

FIG. 9-8 A pulsion diverticulum has a narrow neck and is not easily explored with an endoscope, frequently because either it is filled with ingesta or the scope is too flexible.

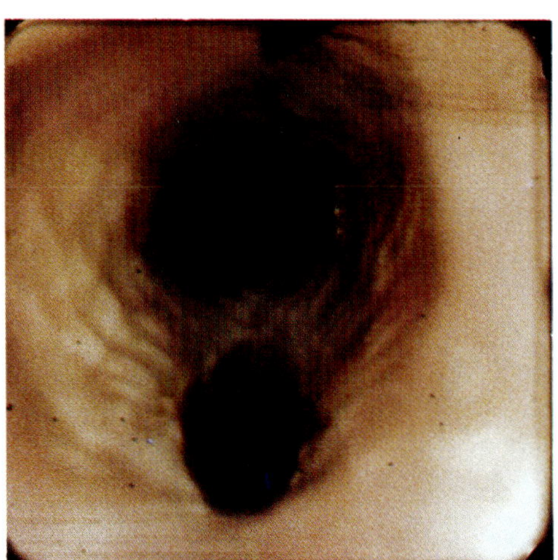

FIG. 9-9 A fistula may be difficult to identify endoscopically because the esophagus is difficult to dilate. Air introduced through the endoscope usually escapes through a fistula of any size. This fistula is the result of dehiscence of an esophagotomy.

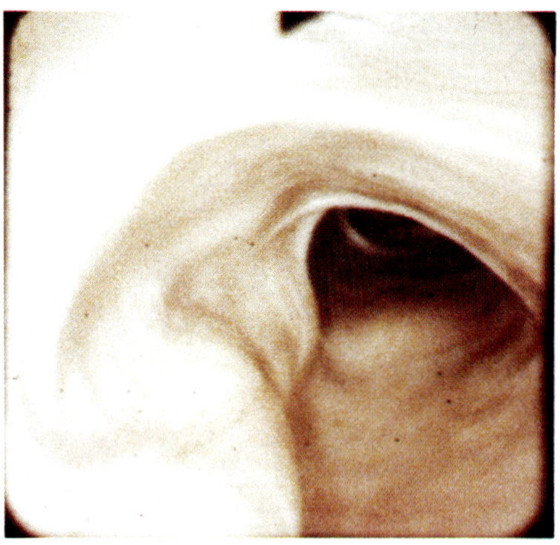

FIG. 9-10 Megaesophagus usually requires lavage and/or suction of the lumen before endoscopy can be completed. This foal has a normal lumen diameter at the cardia but did not require insufflation of the lumen for this examination because air was not being cleared from the esophagus after lavage.

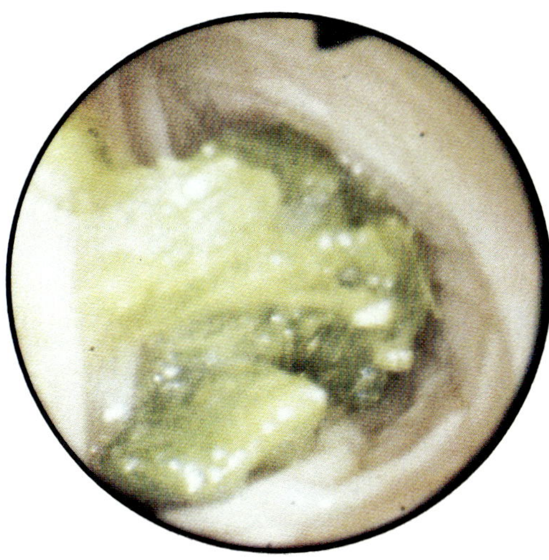

FIG. 9-11 Endoscopy of an impacted esophagus, which usually appears simply as green ingesta and needs to be cleared through lavage before the lumen can be evaluated.

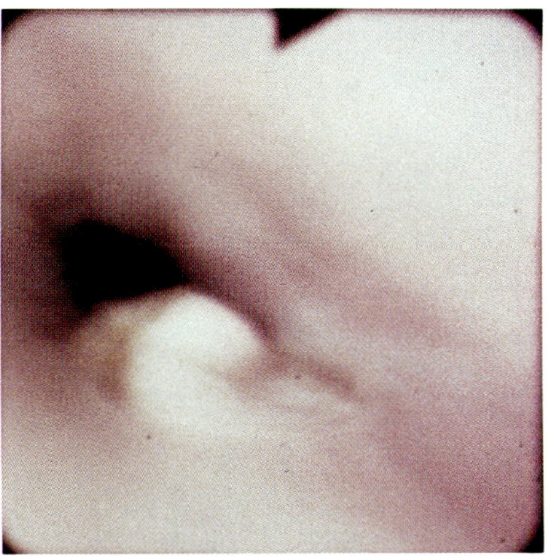

FIG. 9-12 Rupture of the esophagus can be difficult to assess endoscopically because phlegmon in the neck will compress the esophagus and limit movement of the endoscope.

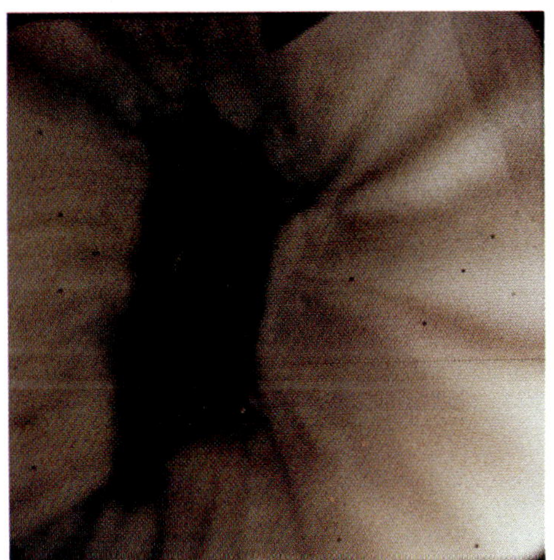

FIG. 9-13 Circumferential mucosal ulceration following feed impaction.

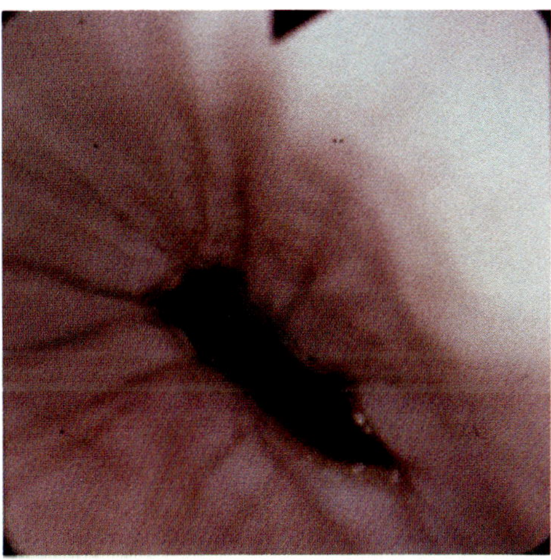

FIG. 9-14 Stricture formation resulting from circumferential ulceration (photograph taken two weeks after Fig 9-13).

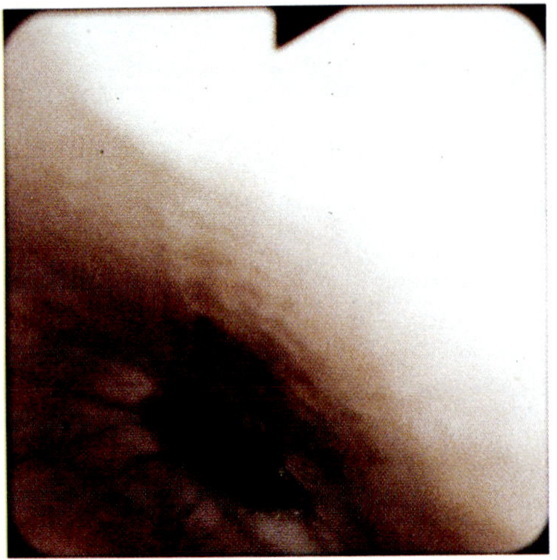

FIG. 9-15 Stricture formation (photo taken four weeks after Fig. 9-13) that resulted in reobstruction.

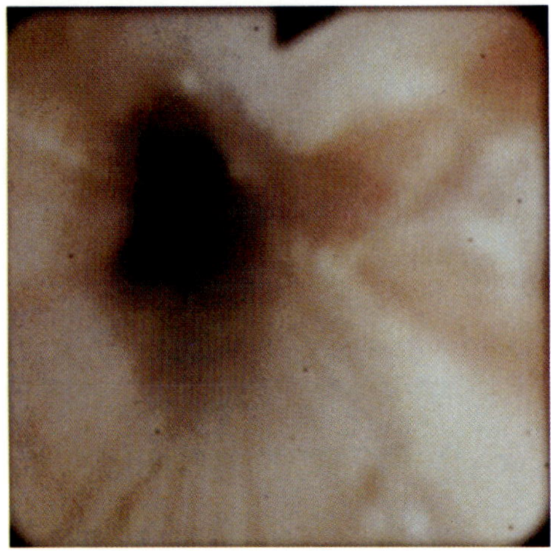

FIG. 9-16 Longitudinal mucosal ulceration following feed impaction that produced 48 hours of odynophagia.

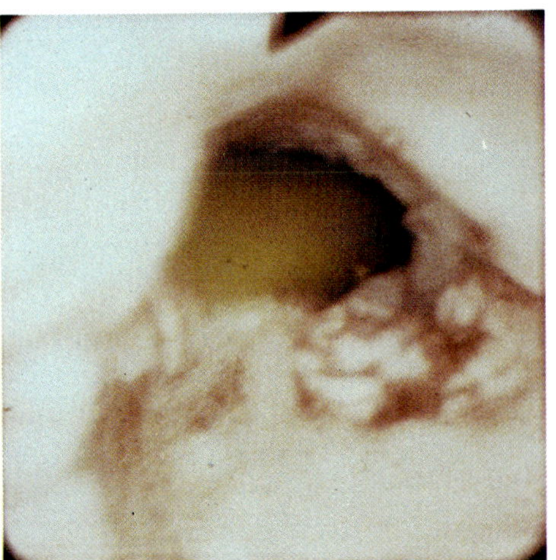

FIG. 9-17 Mucosal ulceration proximal to an esophagostomy tube resulting from ingestion of bedding (wood chips).

Chapter 10

STOMACH

PETER ADAMSON AND MICHAEL J. MURRAY

Endoscopic examination of the stomach in the standing foal and adult horse is routinely performed where appropriate equipment is available. The procedure is relatively quick and easy, due in part to a better understanding of endoscopic techniques and the recent availability of instruments of suitable length.[1] Endoscopy is an accepted method for the diagnosis of upper gastrointestinal tract disease in the horse.

STANDING PROCEDURE: ADULT HORSE AND FOAL

The procedure is similar for adults and foals. The following instruments are required: fiberscope (2 to 3 m in length for adults, and 1.1 to 2.0 M in length for foals, suction, insufflation, biopsy forceps, and lubricant (water-soluble, medical grade). For adult horses, four people are ideal: a leader to control the endoscope head (endoscopist); one to pass the endoscope through a the horse's nostril; one to support and tend equipment; and one to tend the head and twitch. For foals, again four people are needed; one endoscopist; two people to restrain the foal; and one person to pass the endoscope through a the horse's nostril.

Patients should be fasted before gastroscopy according to the following:

AGE	FASTING TIME
Young foals eating minimal solids	Fasting not necessary
Young suckling foals (on solids)	6 to 10 hours
Weanlings	6 to 10 hours
Yearlings and adults	10 to 12 hours

Occasionally, up to 24 hours of fasting is required to ensure gastric emptying.

Appropriate physical and chemical restraint is essential. Weanlings and older horses should be restrained in suitable horse stocks. Foals less than 20 days old can usually be restrained by one or two competent individuals. Older foals and horses may require chemical restraint. Xylazine (0.5 to 0.8 mg/kg of body weight) intravenously, 5 to 10 minutes before commencing the procedure, is satisfactory. A nasal twitch is used as required.

Technique and routine anatomical survey

The lubricated endoscope is passed through a nostril to the dorsal pharynx. Passage of the endoscope through the nasal turbinates can cause the patient to object, but once it is past the turbinates most patients settle down.

The endoscope tip is directed dorsally to the arytenoids and gently advanced, after the swallow reflex is initiated, to enter the cricopharyngeal sphincter region. A stream of water injected through the biopsy channel will induce the swallow reflex.

Resistance at the cricopharyngeal sphincter can cause retroversion of the endoscope with displacement rostral and into the oral cavity if the instrument is advanced (Fig. 10-1). It is important that the endoscopist communicate clearly with the individual passing the endoscope so that the swallow reflex and endoscope advancement are well coordinated. With video endoscopy this is easier because both can observe the endoscopic image.

A momentary loss of visibility occurs as the viewing objective passes the cricopharyngeal sphincter. As the instrument traverses the esophagus, insufflation aids the passage and view. Peristaltic contractions along the esophagus may make advancement of the endoscope difficult, in which case the contraction should be allowed to pass before advancing the endoscope. *Do not advance an endoscope without visibility.*

The entrance to the cardia from the esophagus can be recognized by an oblique cleft (Fig. 10-2). At the entrance to the cardia the endoscopist should assess whether (1) there is any mucosal inflammation present, (2) the entrance is properly closed, and (3) there is gastroesophageal reflux occurring.

As the endoscope is advanced through the short cardiac canal into the stomach, the walls press firmly over the objective, causing a "red out" and a momentary loss of visibility.

The important landmarks to recognize are the entrance to the cardia, the saccus cecus, the margo plicatus, the glandular and nonglandular rugae, the gastric pillar (lesser curvature), the cardiac orifice on the gastric side, and the pyloric region and sphincter (Fig. 10-3).

Almost instantly the stomach can be viewed. Rugae in the fundic nonglandular and glandular areas may be seen, along with some-

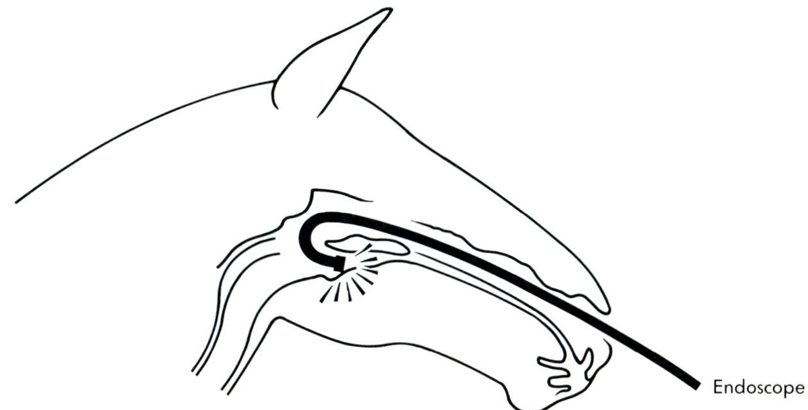

FIG. 10-1 Diagrammatic sagittal section of a horse's head illustrating how the tip of the endoscope can be deflected rostrally into the oral cavity where severe damage by the horse's teeth can occur.

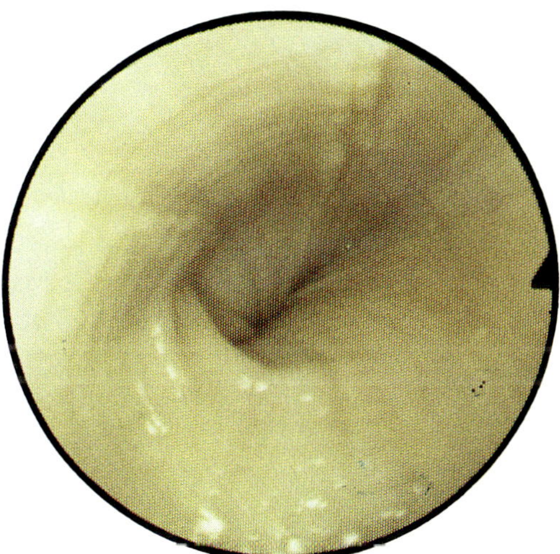

FIG. 10-2 Endoscopic view of the distal esophagus just proximal to the entrance of the cardia, which appears as an oblique cleft.

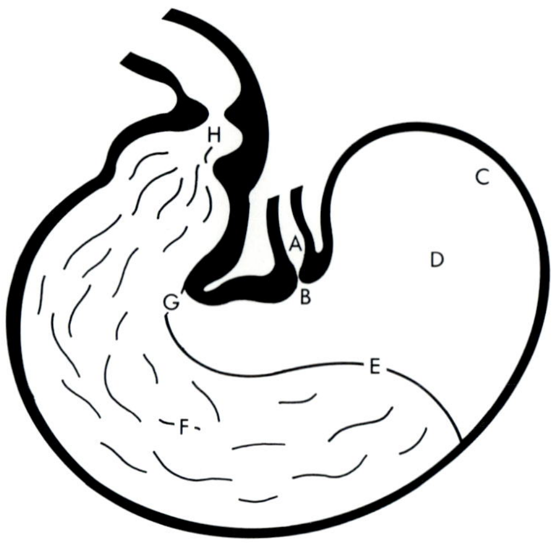

FIG. 10-3 Diagrammatic cross-section of the equine stomach, illustrating the entrance to the cardia *(A);* the cardiac orifice on the gastric side *(B);* saccus cecus *(C);* non-glandular fundus *(D);* margo plicatus *(E);* glandular fundus *(F);* lesser curvature *(G);* and pyloric region *(H).*

food material and a variable fluid lake in the distance. The endoscope objective lies just beyond the gastric cardiac orifice (Fig. 10-4).

Room air is insufflated until a luminal view is obtained, reducing rugal folds by distention and helping to orient the viewer. The mucosal surface should be rinsed with water to remove food material from the surface. Flushing with suction helps to clear the viewing objective and reduce fluid buildup, but will tend to collapse the stomach and enhance rugae formation. Disorientation and frustration can overwhelm beginners at this stage. If disorientation occurs, insufflate the stomach and reorient.

"Red outs" and "white outs" occur when the endoscope contacts the mucosal surfaces and obliterates the forward view. When this occurs, relax, withdraw slightly, clear the viewing objective, insufflate the stomach, and reorient. Occasionally, foreign material cannot be cleaned from the objective by flushing and suction; withdraw the endoscope and gently clean the objective manually. Removing the endoscope tip to the distal esophagus and flushing water through the biopsy channel will often clear the objective.

By directing the viewing objective dorsally and to the horse's right, the squamous fundus and saccus cecus can be seen (Figs. 10-5 and 10-6). By directing the viewing objective ventrally, the squamous fundus, margo plicatus, and glandular fundus of the right side of the stomach between the lesser and greater curvatures can be seen (Fig. 10-7) by directing the viewing objective toward the horse's left. The caudal portion and left caudal portion of the stomach can be viewed (Fig. 10-8).

The mucosal surface of the lesser curvature lies immediately ventral to the cardia, and, in adult horses, can be examined with 5 to 10 cm of the endoscope protruding through the gastric cardiac orifice

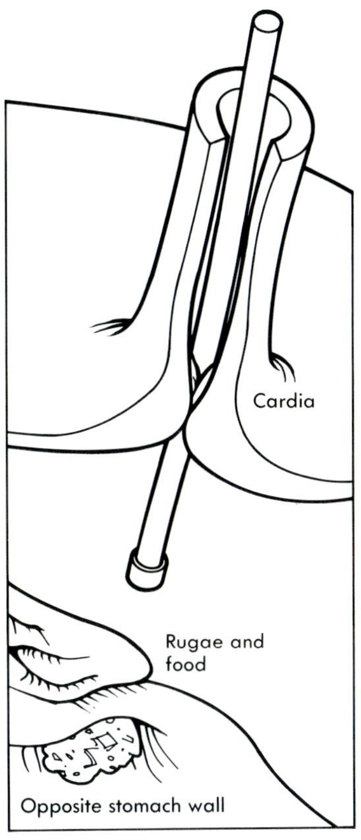

FIG. 10-4 **Diagram illustrating the position of the endoscope** upon initial entry into the undistended stomach.

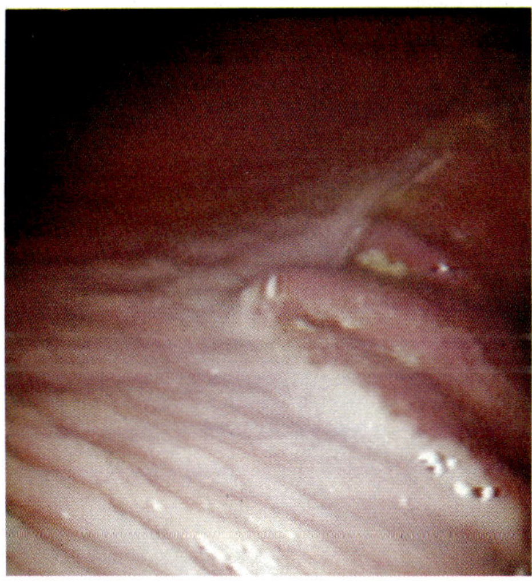

FIG. 10-5 **Endoscopic view of the right portion of the gastric fundus.** The squamous, or non-glandular, portion is to the lower left of the photograph, and the glandular portion is to the right of the photograph.

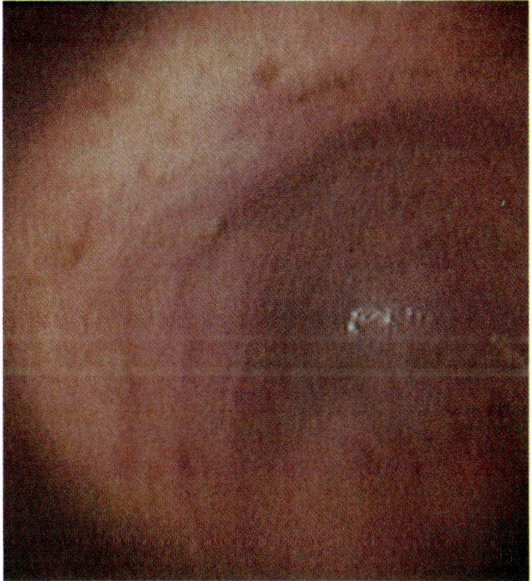

FIG. 10-6 **Endoscopic view of the dorsal portion of the equine stomach,** the saccus caecus. The saccus caecus is a dorsal out-pouching of the stomach.

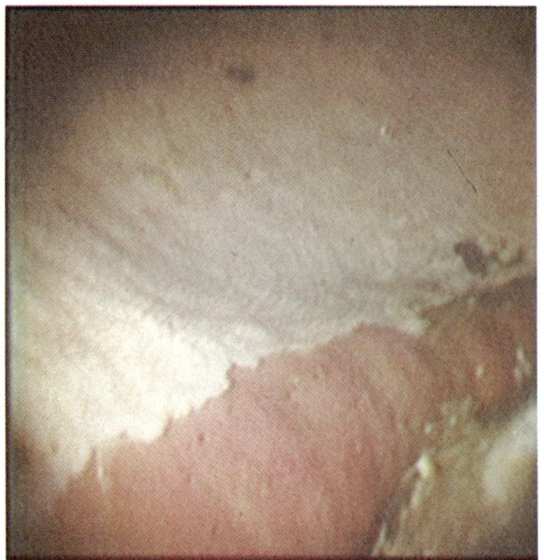

FIG. 10-7 Endoscopic view of the right portion of the gastric fundus, illustrating the irregular border, the margo plicatus, between the white squamous (top) and pink glandular (bottom) portions of the fundus.

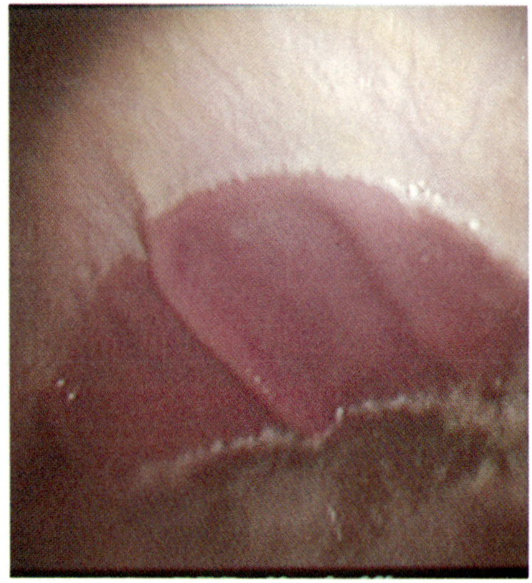

FIG. 10-8 Caudal portion of the equine stomach along the greater curvature. The squamous mucosal surface is at the top and glandular mucosal surface at the bottom of the photograph. Gastric fluid, a normal amount that is present after withholding feed for 12 to 14 hours, can be seen at the extreme bottom of the photograph.

and directed ventrally and to the horse's left (Figs. 10-9 and 10-10). The caudal pyloric antrum can now be viewed. Anatomically, the pyloric sphincter lies cranial and ventral to a ridge (gastric pillar) formed by the lesser curvature and is just out of sight.

The squamous fundus and margo plicatus should be examined carefully, using as aids a combination of tip deflection and endoscope head rotation. Careful examination of the entire margo plicatus is essential because it is the site of most ulcerative lesions in horses and may be the site for early squamous cell carcinoma development in older horses.

In adult horses, the majority of lesions occur in the region of the squamous fundus and margo plicatus along the greater curvature. Careful examination is advised in this region.[6]

The area of the glandular mucosal surface that can be examined will depend on the amount of food and fluid retained after fasting and on the degree of distention achieved through insufflation. Approximately 60% of the glandular mucosal surface can be examined in fasted horses and young foals eating minimal solids (Fig. 10-11).

At this point, the deflecting section of the endoscope should be repositioned to view the margo plicatus in the region of the greater curvature.

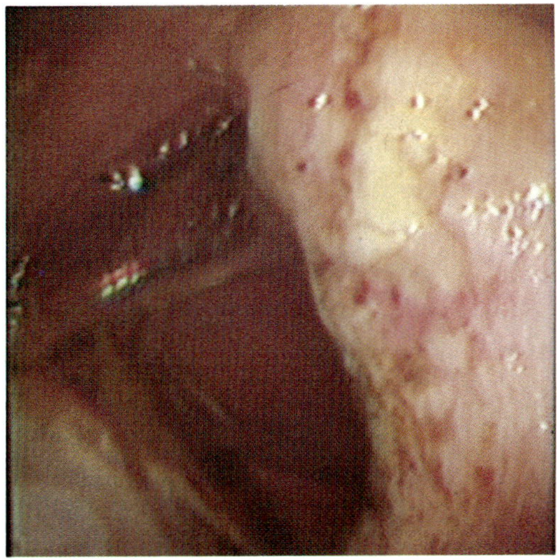

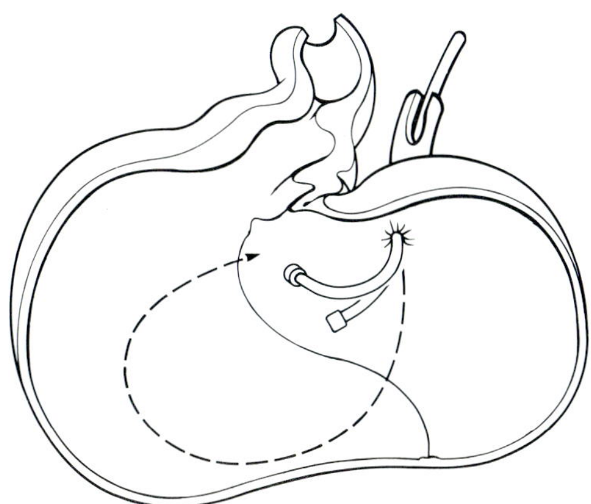

FIG. 10-9 **The lesser curvature,** or
gastric pillar, is at the right of the
photograph. There is moderate
ulceration present in the squamous
mucosal surface of the lesser curvature.
This image is angled approximately 45°
to the left, and fluid in the antral portion
of the stomach can be seen at the lower
left of the photograph.

FIG. 10-10 **Diagram illustrating the
positions of the endoscope objective**
that are required to observe the lesser
curvature. The broken line indicates the
route the endoscope travels around the
stomach to view the lesser curvature
end-on. The relation between the length
of the endoscope and the size of the
foal/horse will determine which method
of viewing is used to observe the lesser
curvature and cardiac orifice.

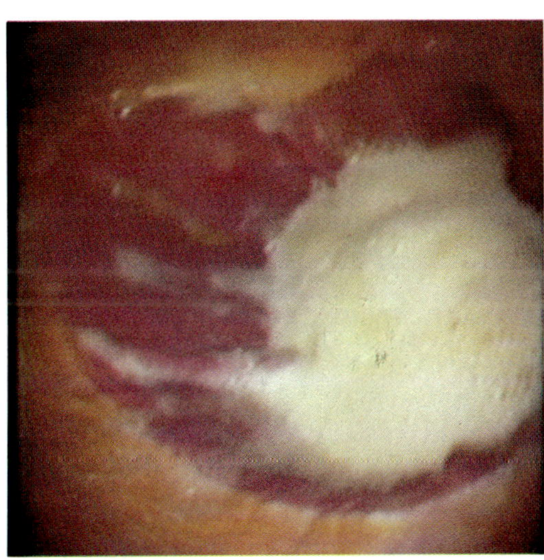

FIG. 10-11 **The ventral portion of
the stomach** as viewed from the right
dorsal portion of the stomach. The
caudal portion of the stomach, along the
greater curvature, is at the left of the
photograph, and the pyloric antrum and
outflow tract is at the upper right. A
puddle of frothy fluid is in the glandular
fundic and antral portions of the
stomach. The squamous mucosal surface
has a yellow-orange coloration, resulting
from keratinization of the squamous
mucosa caused by acid injury.

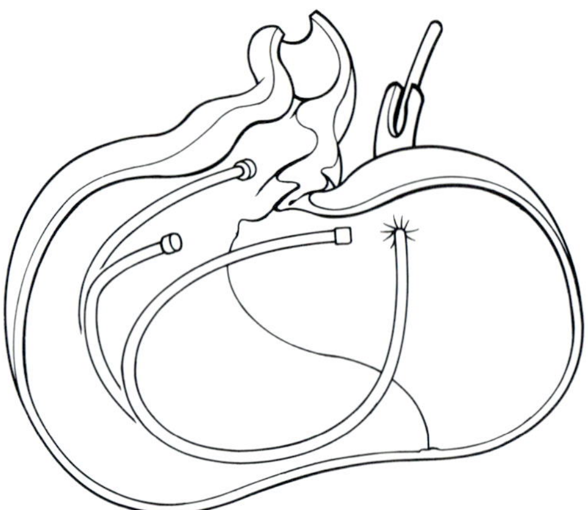

FIG. 10-12 Diagram illustrating the route taken by the endoscope to visualize the cardiac region, the lesser curvature, and pyloric outflow tract.

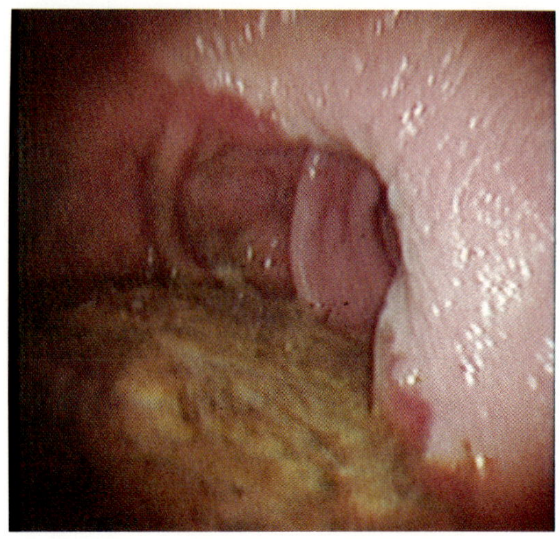

FIG. 10-13 The lesser curvature (right) and antral region of the equine stomach, viewed with the endoscope advanced around the greater curvature, as illustrated in Fig. 10-12. Feed material in the antral region is seen at the lower left of the photograph.

Next, the endoscope is advanced toward the greater curvature, with the viewing objective turning away from the nonglandular fundus, and advanced along the greater curvature. The aim is to travel around the greater curvature and not straight ahead (Fig. 10-12). The endoscope forms a loop within the stomach that, combined with viewing objective deflection toward the gastric pillar (Fig. 10-13), allows examination of the lesser curvature and gastric cardiac orifice (Fig. 10-14).

The gastric pillar is examined end-on. The margo plicatus and gastric cardiac orifice should be closely examined by gently advancing the looped endoscope.

If the endoscope is long enough, the viewing objective is directed toward the axis of the pyloric antrum, and the antrum and pylorus are examined from a distance. With the aid of gastric contractions, the endoscope can be advanced to the pylorus and into the duodenal ampulla. Entering the pyloric area is not always possible and may require several attempts. The viewing objective has to be directed so that the antrum and pyloric rim are visible as the endoscope is advanced. The endoscope objective will frequently impinge on the stomach wall, causing the "red out" phenomenon. The viewing objective has to be cleared frequently and the endoscope withdrawn to reorient as necessary. In foals with absent or weak gastric motility, the endoscope often cannot be advanced to

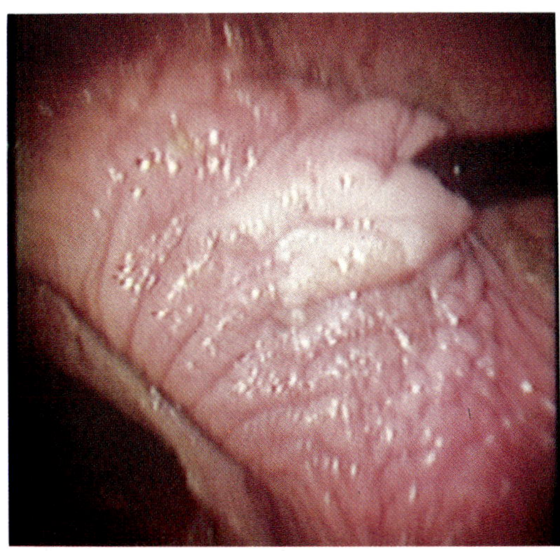

FIG. 10-14 Lesser curvature and cardiac orifice. Note the endoscope insertion tube in the cardiac orifice.

the pylorus. In these cases, the endoscope will coil up in the stomach without the objective advancing.

Contractions of the antrum, pyloric canal, and pyloric ring should be carefully observed (Figs. 10-15 and 10-16). Endoscope rotation and tip deflection allow complete examination of the area, excluding areas obscured by a fluid lake or food material in the pyloric antrum.

When possible, the duodenal ampulla should be examined for evidence of inflammation and for ulceration (Figs. 10-17 and 10-18) and bile reflux. In some cases, the endoscope can be advanced farther to examine the duodenum and opening of the common bile duct.

On completion of the procedure, the endoscope is slowly withdrawn and all structures again closely observed.

In cases in which the endoscope is too short to reach the pylorus, examination of the animal under general anesthesia and in lateral recumbency may permit observation of this area. This technique has been useful in large weanlings and smaller yearlings.

RECUMBENT PROCEDURE: THE FOAL UNDER GENERAL ANESTHESIA

Endoscopic examination of the stomach in foals under general anesthesia allows a complete and thorough examination of the entire gastric mucosa. The technique is useful for research purposes and in cases in which patients are resistant to the standing procedure. It is particularly useful when food obliterates adequate examination of the gastric pillar and pyloric antrum. The major disadvantage of the endoscopic technique is the additional stress caused by general anes-

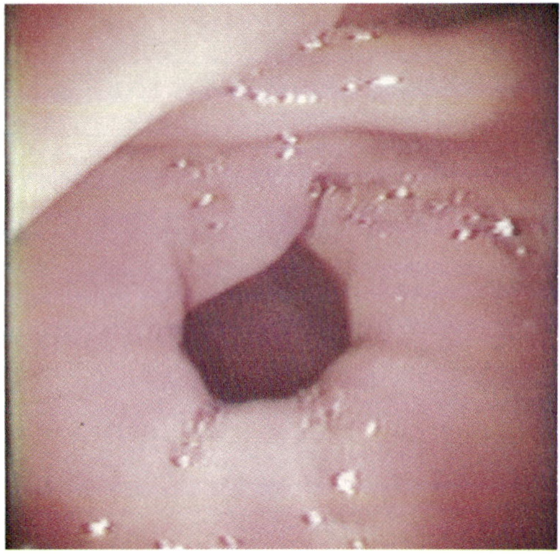

FIG. 10-15 **Pyloric sphincter** in the open position.

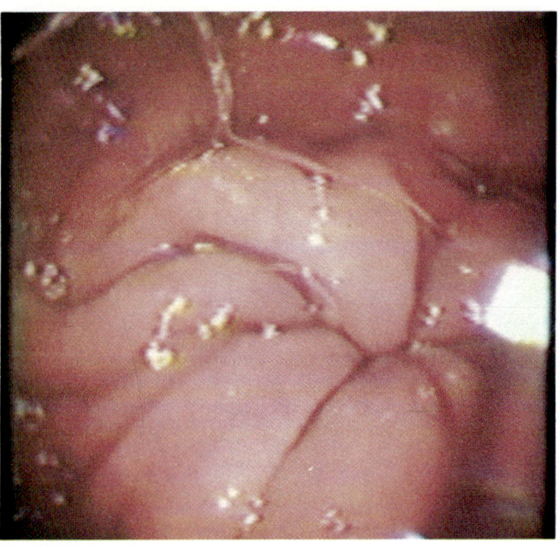

FIG. 10-16 **Pyloric sphincter** in the closed position.

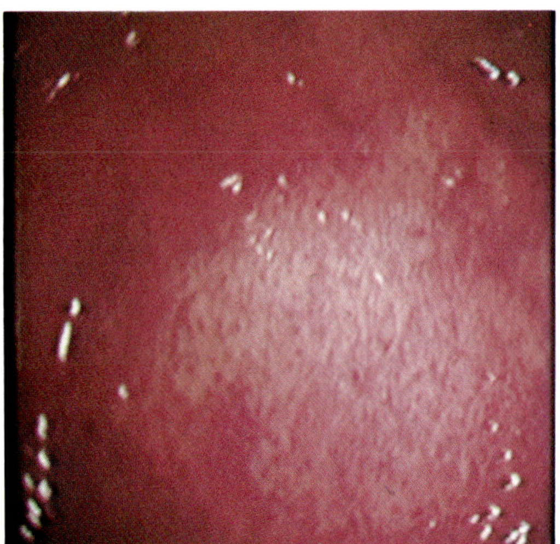

FIG. 10-17 **View of the duodenal ampulla** in a foal with duodenitis. There is diffuse hyperemia of the mucosal surface, which should appear pale pink.

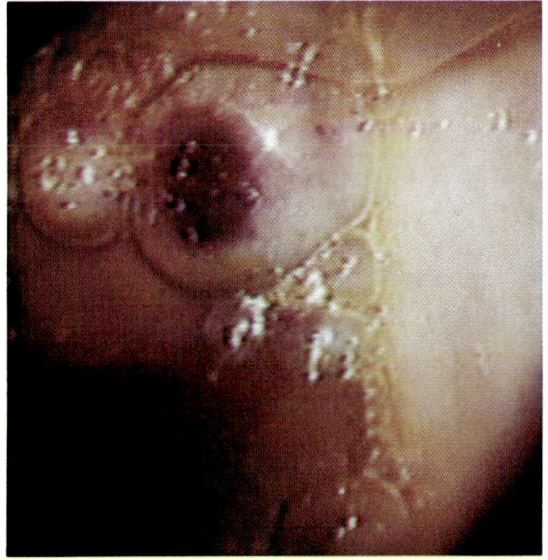

FIG. 10-18 **View of the duodenal ampulla** in a foal with chronic diarrhea and anemia. A 2 cm diameter bleeding ulcer is in the middle of the photograph.

thesia. In most foals the procedure can be performed under sedation with xylazine in combination with diazepam or butorphanol.

The technique is similar for weanlings and foals and uses the same equipment as for the standing procedure in addition to suitable inhalant anesthetic equipment.

Four people are needed: one endoscopist; one to pass endoscope through the horse's nostril; one to reposition the patient, and one to supervise anesthesia.

All solid foodstuffs are removed 10 hours before the examination, but access to the dam and water is allowed right up to the time of examination. Do not muzzle the foal because muzzling appears to delay gastric emptying.

Appropriate chemical restraint of the mare is advisable before separating the foal. General anesthesia is induced using a protocol of choice allowing for 45 to 60 minutes of anesthesia.

Technique and routine anatomical survey

The anesthetized or sedated foal is positioned in right lateral recumbency using appropriate padding. The endoscopist should be comfortably seated in front of the foal's head on an adjustable stool.

The well-lubricated endoscope is passed through a nostril to the dorsal pharynx with care taken not to damage the nasal turbinates. The endoscope is directed dorsally to the arytenoids and gently advanced through the cricopharyngeal sphincter region, using insufflation. The important landmarks to recognize are the same as those for the standing procedure (Fig. 10-4).

When the endoscope objective lies just beyond the gastric cardiac orifice, insufflate until a luminal view is obtained, reducing the rugae by distention of the gastric lumen. A fluid lake often accumulates around the gastric cardiac orifice (to the endoscopist's left) initially obliterating the view. This can appear as a "yellowish green out." Using suction at this time reduces this fluid lake. The suction channel is blocked easily because of solid food fragments and may be rendered ineffectual for the remainder of the procedure until cleaning. The glandular and nonglandular fundus and the margo plicatus are examined by using the viewing objective deflection and endoscope head rotation. The endoscope is advanced toward the margo plicatus and the viewing objective directed away from the nonglandular fundus. The glandular fundus of the greater curvature, the entrance to the pyloric antrum, and the region of the lesser curvature are examined.

In the well-distended empty stomach the endoscope can often be directed into the pyloric antrum and advanced toward the pyloric sphincter while the patient is in right lateral recumbency. If the pyloric antrum and gastric pillar are obscured from view by a food material bolus firmly in position, or by fluid, the patient is rolled

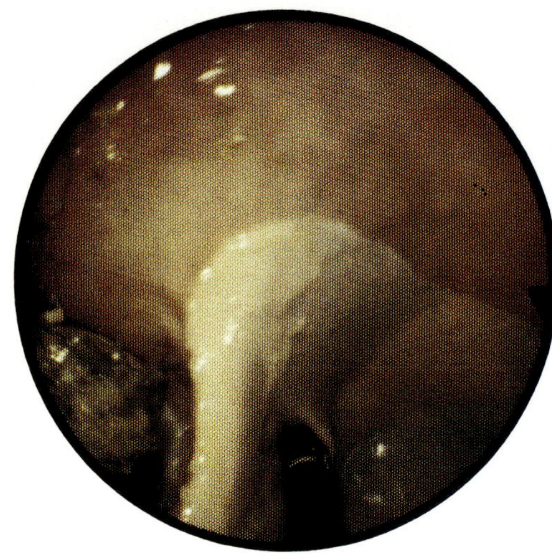

FIG. 10-19 View of a portion of the glandular fundus, lesser curvature, and cardia as observed in a foal in right lateral recumbency. Feed material, at the lower right of the photograph, is in a portion of the stomach that is dependent because of positioning in right lateral recumbency.

into dorsal recumbency. The bolus will be dislodged from beneath the gastric pillar and come to lie in the region of the pyloric antrum.

The looped endoscope is advanced toward the gastric pillar and the margo plicatus examined for evidence of lesions (Fig. 10-19). The gastric cardiac orifice is examined for evidence of inflammation. Viewing objective deflection and endoscope head rotation are necessary to adequately view these structures.

In some cases, rolling the patient into left lateral recumbency helps passage of the endoscope into the pyloric antrum and through the pyloric sphincter. Additionally, antral food boluses are dislodged into the saccus cecus region, allowing adequate visualization of the pyloric antrum.

On completion of the procedure, withdraw the endoscope slowly and closely observe all structures again. Deflate the stomach by using suction before complete withdrawal.

ABNORMALITIES AND LESIONS OF THE STOMACH

The appearance and location of lesions in the stomach vary with the age of the horse. In neonatal foals, lesions in the squamous mucosa adjacent to the margo plicatus along the greater curvature of the stomach develop as early as 2 days of age. These lesions begin as a yellow, crusty area with some desquamation of squamous epithelium (Fig. 10-20), and in a few days can progress to one or more areas of ulceration (Fig. 10-21). They occur in 50% of normal thoroughbred foals and possibly in foals of other breeds.[6,7]

Epithelial desquamation, which is the shedding of the superficial layers of the squamous epithelium of the stomach, occurs in the majority of young foals.[6,7] This desquamation appears as flakes of

TABLE 10-1 Conditions of the equine stomach which may be diagnosed endoscopically

CONDITION	CLINICAL SIGNS
Gastric ulcers	
Foal (Figs. 10-20 to 10-26)	Variable depending on severity; includes colic, bruxism, excessive salivation, diarrhea, and poor growth
Adults (Figs. 10-27 to 10-29)	Often vague; poor performance; weight loss; low-grade colic; "sour" attitude
Gasterophilus larvae (Fig. 10-30)	Often no signs; possible ill thrift
Draschia larvae (Fig. 10-31)	None
Pyloric stenosis (Fig. 10-32)	Colic; ill thrift, plus signs of gastric ulceration
Squamous cell carcinoma (Fig. 10-33)	Chronic weight loss

tissue on the squamous mucosal surface (Fig. 10-22) or as large sheets of tissue separating from the dorsal fundus toward the margo plicatus (Fig. 10-23).

Lesions in the glandular mucosa occur in very few normal asymptomatic foals[6,7], but are common in foals with typical signs of gastroduodenal ulceration.[3] These lesions are often not as dramatic in appearance as squamous lesions and appear as either linear lesions or as focal defects in the glandular mucosa (Figs. 10-24 and 10-25). The glandular mucosa normally appears very smooth and velvety. Inflammation of the glandular mucosa, without discrete ulceration, can appear as a roughened or reticulated pattern on the mucosa. Passage of the endoscope to the pylorus may reveal ulceration surrounding the pylorus in cases with duodenal ulceration.

In older foals, lesions can be observed in the squamous mucosa of the lesser curvature and surrounding the cardia (Fig. 10-26). These lesions can be severe and have been associated with duodenal ulceration and nonobstructive gastric emptying disorders.[4] Lesions also can be observed in the squamous fundus and adjacent to the margo plicatus on the right side of the stomach in older foals.

The distribution of ulcerative or erosive lesions in adult horses is most frequent in the squamous mucosa adjacent to the margo plicatus (Fig. 10-27), the squamous fundus (Fig. 10-28), and the lesser curvature (Fig. 10-9).[5] There is hemorrhage associated with these lesions in approximately one third of cases. The severity of lesions varies but is greater in horses with clinical signs that are associated with gastric lesions.[5] Horses with several lesions, or bleeding lesions, should be treated, preferably, with histamine type II receptor antagonists.[2] Lesions occur infrequently in the glandular mucosa of adult horses (Fig. 10-29) and are usually present in conjunction with lesions of the squamous mucosa.

Gasterophilus larvae can frequently be seen, either singly or in groups (Fig. 10-30). Lesions attributed to *Draschia (Habronema) megastoma* are also common. These are either at the margo plicatus or in the glandular region (Fig. 10-31). Occasional additional lesions include pyloric stenosis (Fig. 10-32) and squamous cell carcinoma (Fig. 10-33).

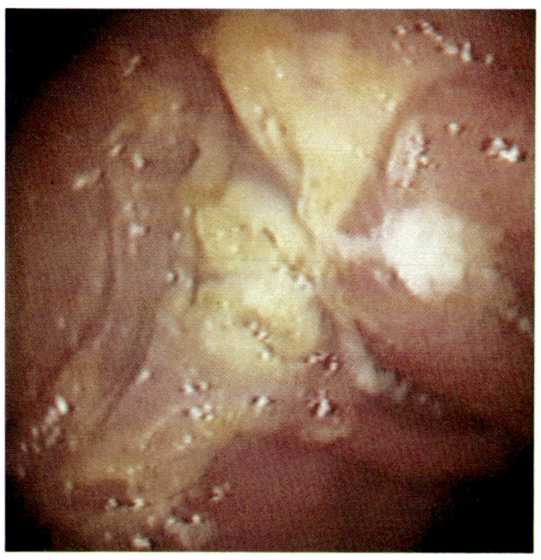

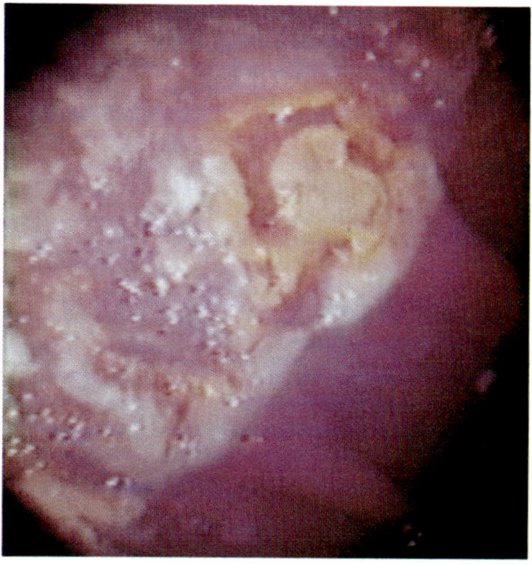

FIG. 10-20 Caudal fundus of a 3-day-old foal, with the squamous portion at the left and the glandular portion at the right of the photograph. At the center of the photograph, two lesions surrounded by a yellow, crusty material can be seen in the squamous mucosa adjacent to the margo plicatus. This is the typical appearance of lesions, as they begin to form, that are observed in 50% of normal neonatal foals.

FIG. 10-21 Similar view as in Fig. 10-20, from a 5-day-old foal that has more extensive ulceration of the squamous mucosa adjacent to the margo plicatus.

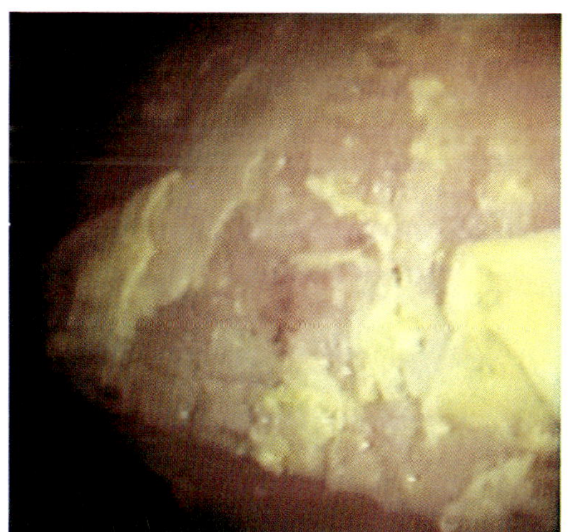

FIG. 10-22 Similar view as in Figures 10-20, 10-21, illustrating the flaky appearance of desquamating squamous epithelium in a 14-day-old foal.

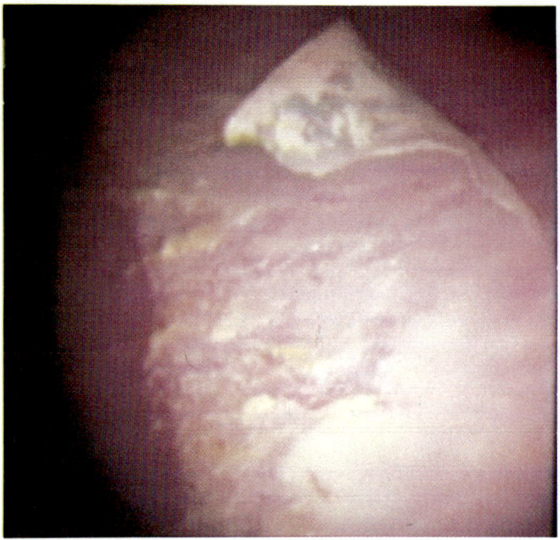

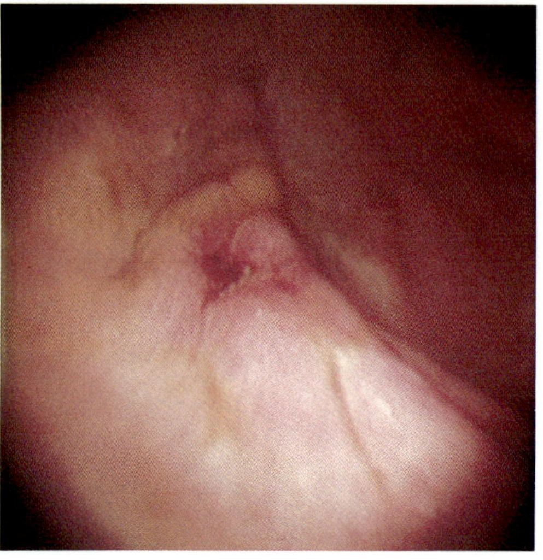

FIG. 10-23   **A large sheet of desquamating epithelium** is seen to be separating from the underlying squamous mucosa toward the margo plicatus, at the left of the photograph.

FIG. 10-24   **Glandular mucosal ulcer** in a 3-day-old septic foal. The ulcer is on a rugal fold and has a hemorrhagic center.

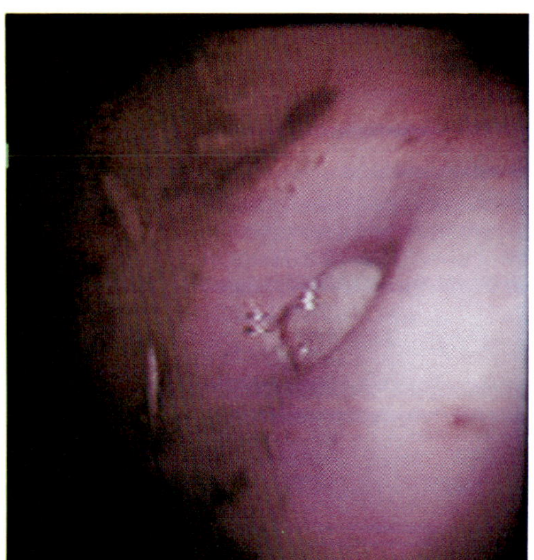

FIG. 10-25   **Deep ulcer** in the glandular mucosa at the lesser curvature of a foal with suspected botulism. This lesion extended down to the serosal surface of the stomach.

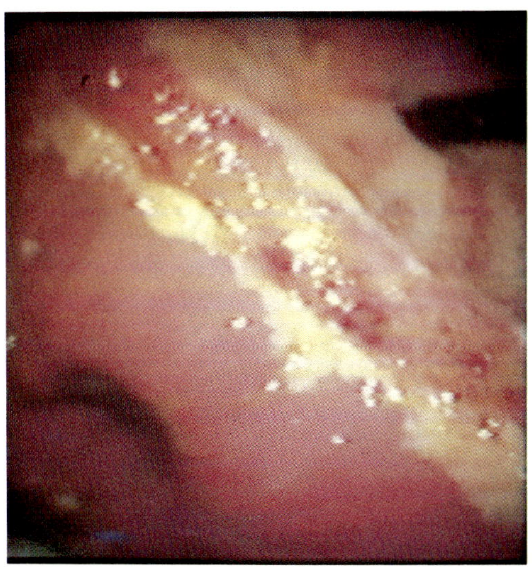

FIG. 10-26 View of the lesser curvature and cardiac region of a weanling foal with chronic diarrhea and a non–obstructive gastric emptying disorder. There is a wide band of ulceration of the squamous mucosa adjacent to the margo plicatus along the lesser curvature, as well as ulceration surrounding the cardia. The endoscope is seen through the cardia at the upper right of the photograph.

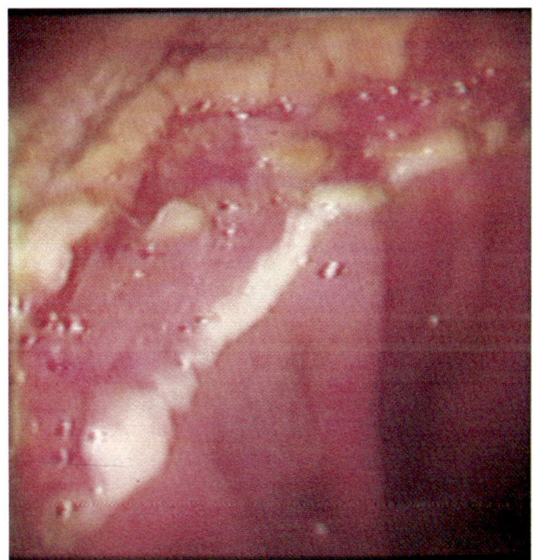

FIG. 10-27 A wide band of severe ulceration of the squamous mucosa adjacent to the margo plicatus along the greater curvature in a 3-year-old Thoroughbred filly. The filly had a poor appetite and was in poor condition; both her appetite and condition improved when she was treated with a histamine type-2 receptor antagonist.

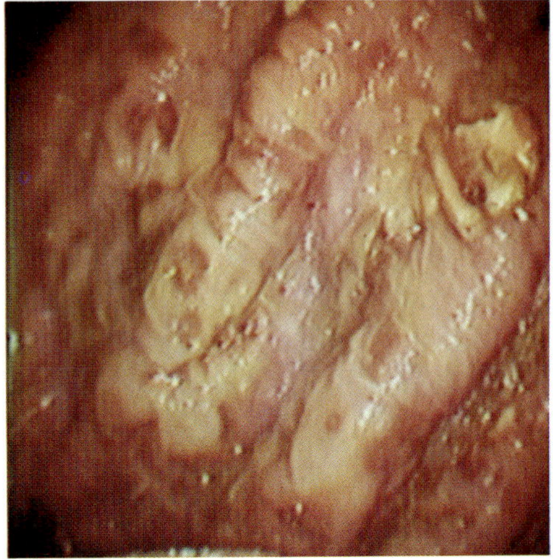

FIG. 10-28 Severe multifocal ulceration of the squamous mucosa of the gastric fundus of a 4-year-old Thoroughbred filly with a poor appetite and poor condition. The appetite improved and the lesions healed after treatment with a histamine type-2 receptor antagonist.

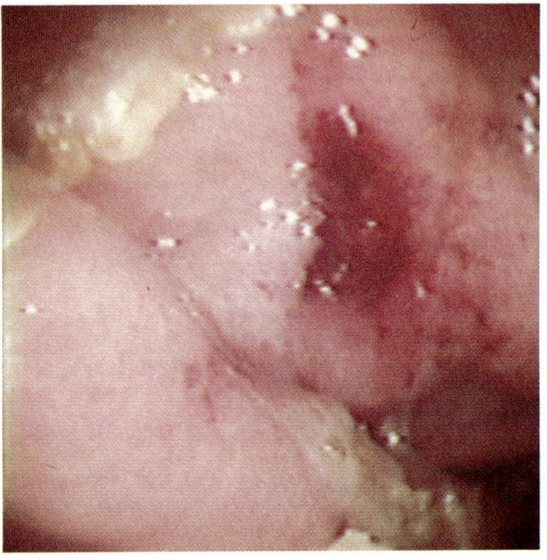

FIG. 10-29 Hemorrhagic ulcer in the glandular mucosa of a 3-year-old Thoroughbred filly.

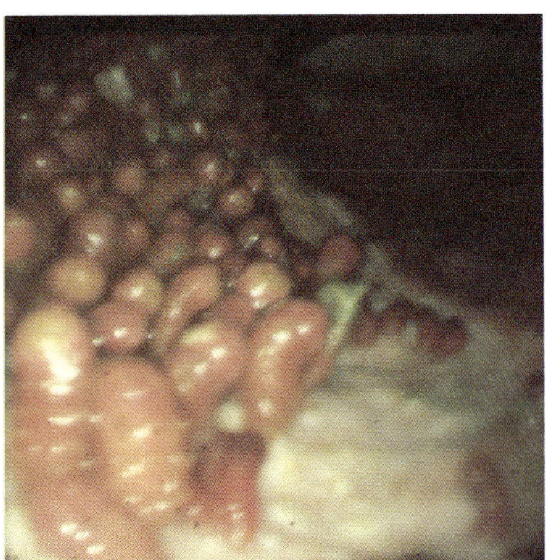

FIG. 10-30 Adult equine stomach with a large number of *Gasterophilus* larvae attached to the mucosa.

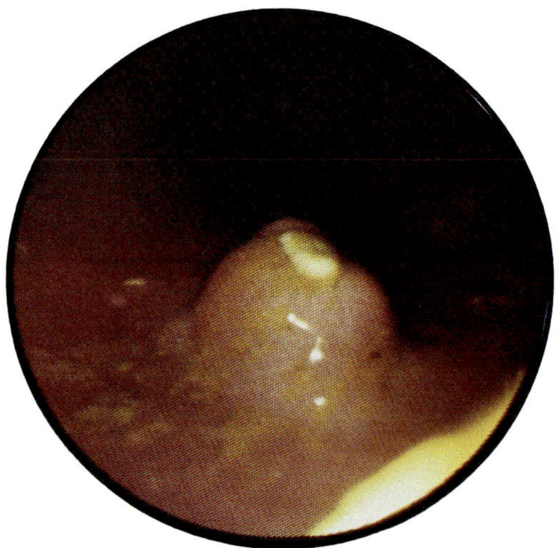

FIG. 10-31 Endoscopic view of a *Draschia megastoma* lesion in the glandular fundus of a horse.

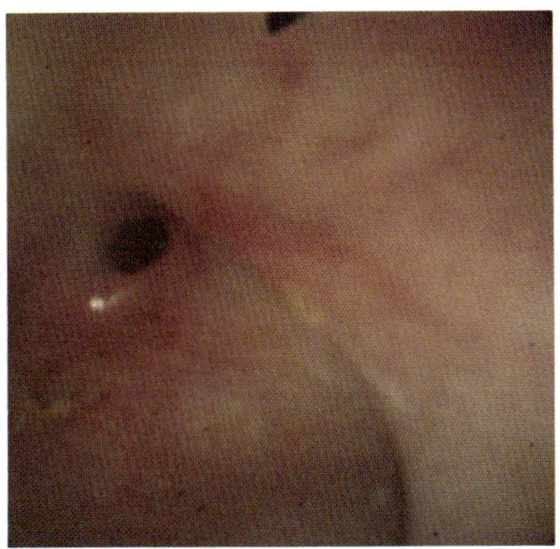

FIG. 10-32 Pyloric region in a foal with pyloric stenosis. The pyloric orifice is small, and failed to dilate any further during observation.

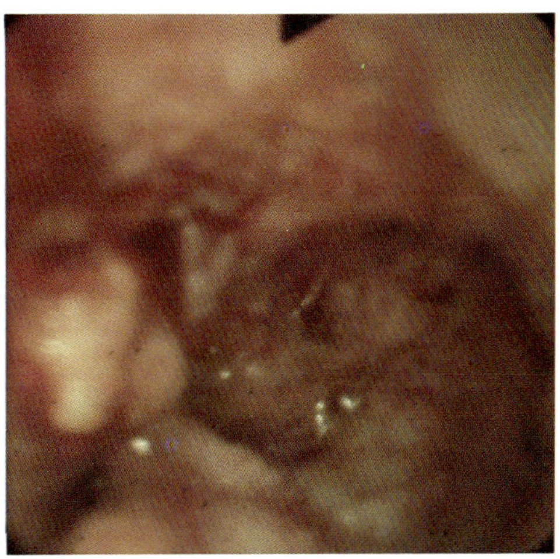

FIG. 10-33 Squamous cell carcinoma of the stomach. The normal anatomy is obscured.

REFERENCES

1. Brown CM, Slocombe RF, and Derksen FJ: Fiberoptic gastroduodenoscopy in the horse, J Am Vet Med Assoc 186:965, 1985.
2. Furr MO and Murray MJ: Treatment of gastric ulcers in horses with histamine type 2 receptor antagonists, Abstracts Third Equine Colic Res Symp 17, 1988.
3. Murray MJ: Endoscopic appearance of gastric lesions in foals: 94 cases (1987-1988), J Am Vet Med Assoc 195: 1135, 1989.
4. Murray MJ: Non-obstructive gastric paresis and gastric ulceration in foals and horses unpublished data, 1989.
5. Murray MJ et al: Gastric ulcers in horses: a comparison of endoscopic findings in horses with and without clinical signs, Equine Vet J (in press) 1989.
6. Murray MJ, Hart J, and Parker GA Equine gastric ulcer syndrome: endoscopic survey of asymptomatic foals, Proc Am Assoc Equine Pract 33, 669, 1987.
7. Murray MJ et al: Prevalence of gastric lesions in normal foals in Ireland and England: an endoscopic survey, Equine Vet J (in press) 1989.

Chapter 11

Duodenum

BENJAMIN J. DARIEN

The incidence of duodenal disease in equine medicine is not well established. In recent years, however, the availability of flexible fiberoptic endoscopes has contributed greatly to the examination and treatment of duodenal disease. Duodenoscopy should be performed only when physical and radiographic examinations have been completed. Signs of gastroduodenal obstruction and/or radiographic evidence of gastric distension (gas and fluid) will prevent viewing of the pyloric antrum and successful duodenoscopy.

The duodenum not only is a repository for peptic ulcer but also may be a harbor for a wide variety of diseases, both primary and secondary. Inflammatory, neoplastic, or infectious diseases are readily identifiable endoscopically, and some may be definitely diagnosed by endoscopic biopsy.

EXAMINATION OF THE DUODENUM

Patient preparation and restraint

Prior to gastroduodenoscopy, the horse should be withheld from feed for at least 24 hours and in some cases up to 48 hours, and from water for at least two hours. To safely perform gastroduodenoscopy, it is imperative that the patient be well restrained because rapid retraction of the endoscope is hindered by the length of the endoscope. The use of restraint stocks, xylazine (0.5 mg/kg of body weight), and a twitch is usually sufficient for most patients. However, the addition of butorphanol tartrate (0.02 mg/kg of body weight) is helpful for the uncooperative patient. The assistance of three people to help with restraint and support of the long scope will facilitate the examination.

Special equipment

Duodenoscopy can be performed in foals that weigh less than 90 kg with a 200 cm endoscope, provided the diameter is sufficiently small (9 to 11 mm) to pass through the ventral meatus without traumatizing the turbinates. Horses heavier than 150 to 200 kg will require an endoscope 275 to 310 cm long. The advantages of the longer scope are increased stability (11 to 13.5 mm in diameter), larger biopsy channel (2.8 mm diameter), and larger field of view with improved optics. Biopsy instruments designed for the larger biopsy channels have a deeper basket and yield more positive histopathologic diagnoses.

Technique

Passage of the endoscope into the duodenum requires that the operator advance the scope along the greater curvature of the stomach until the cardiac orifice and endoscope are viewed. The endoscope is then advanced (while directing the tip away from the cardiac orifice) until the pyloric antrum can be seen (Fig. 11-1). The scope must then be directed into and through the pylorus to the duodenum (Fig. 11-2). It may not be possible to introduce the scope into the duodenum of all horses, and it does take time and patience for the operator to be successful.

NORMAL DUODENAL ANATOMY

The duodenal mucous membrane is soft and velvety. It has a grayish or yellowish-red color and is very vascular (Fig. 11-3). Five to six inches from the pylorus it forms a pouch (the duodenal diverticulum) (Fig. 11-4) in which the pancreatic and hepatic ducts open. On a small papilla nearly opposite this is the termination of the accessory pancreatic duct. A yellow to greenish brown, clear fluid can often be seen in the lumen of the duodenum (Fig. 11-5). This is most likely bile mixed with pancreatic fluid, which can be seen being secreted through the duodenal diverticulum (Fig. 11-6). The duodenal glands are present in the proximal third of the small intestine. Their ducts perforate the muscularis mucosa and the mucous membrane. Active peristalsis is observed during duodenoscopy (Fig. 11-7).

DISEASES OF THE DUODENUM

Duodenoscopy affords the clinician a view of active disease processes in the proximal duodenum (Table 11-1 lists duodenal diseases.). Duodenal ulcers (Fig. 11-8) and parasites (Figs. 11-9 & 11-10) are commonly diagnosed, and, many times, parasites can be seen by looking through the pylorus (Fig. 11-11). Duodenal biopsy (Fig. 11-12) for histopathology and culture, and bile aspiration (Fig. 11-13) for biochemical evaluation and culture can be performed with special equipment directed through the biopsy channel.

TABLE 11-1 Duodenal disease

CONDITION	CLINICAL SIGNS
Ulcer (Fig. 11-8)	Chronic, low grade abdominal pain unresponsive to conventional medical therapy; lethargy; depression; anorexia; adontoprisis; and sialism
Gasterophilus nasalis (Figs. 11-9, 11-10, and 11-11)	Low-grade abdominal pain; anorexia; unthriftiness; poor hair coat; diarrhea

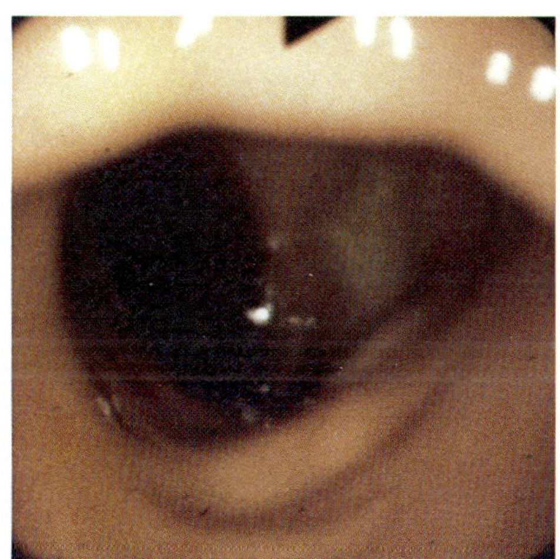

FIG. 11-1 **Duodenum,** seen through the pyloric antrum.

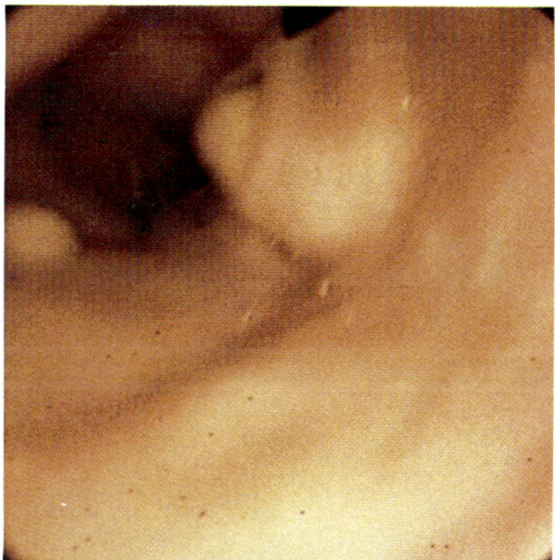

FIG. 11-2 **Gastroscopy,** viewing the duodenal diverticulum.

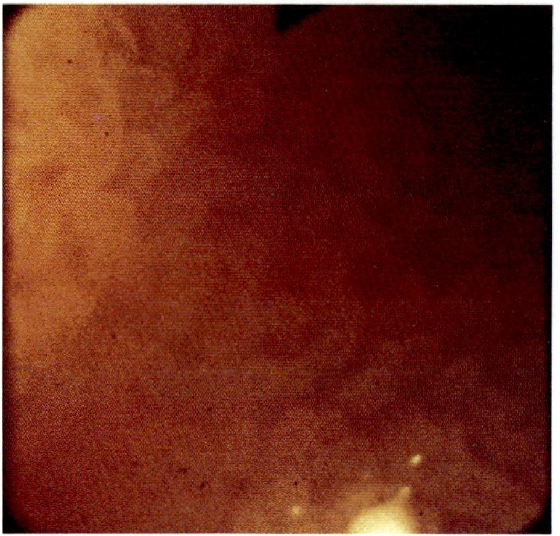

FIG. 11-3   **Close-up view of duodenal mucosa.** Villi are easily identified.

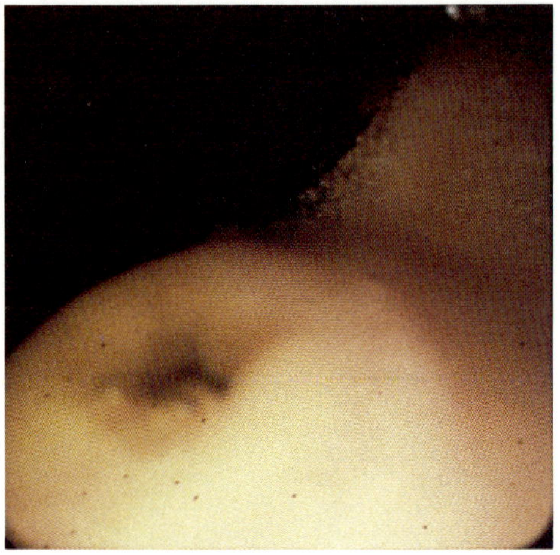

FIG. 11-4   **Duodenal diverticulum.**

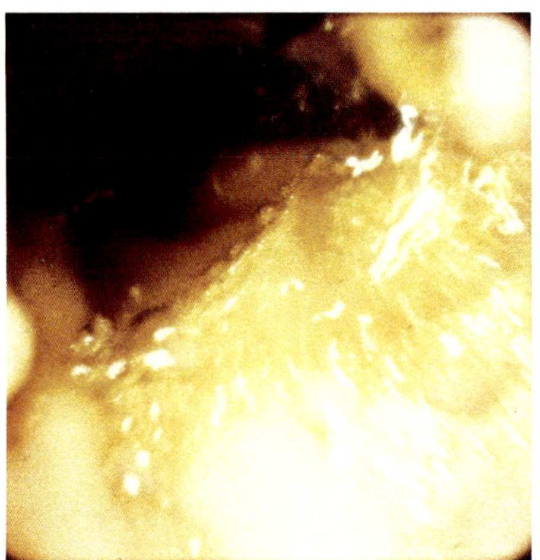

FIG. 11-5   **Lumen of duodenum.** The mucosa is paler than that of the stomach, and clear yellow bile is present.

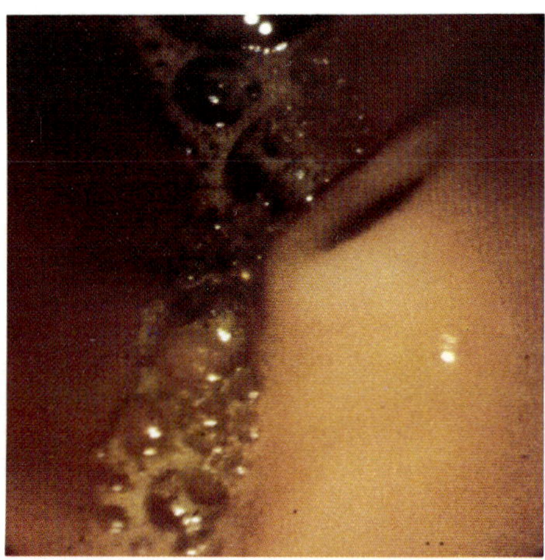

FIG. 11-6   **Bile and pancreatic fluid** being secreted from the duodenal diverticulum.

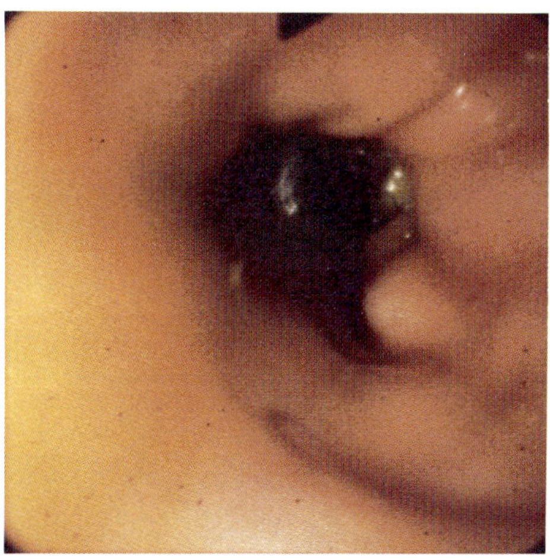

FIG. 11-7 **Duodenum,** active paristalsis.

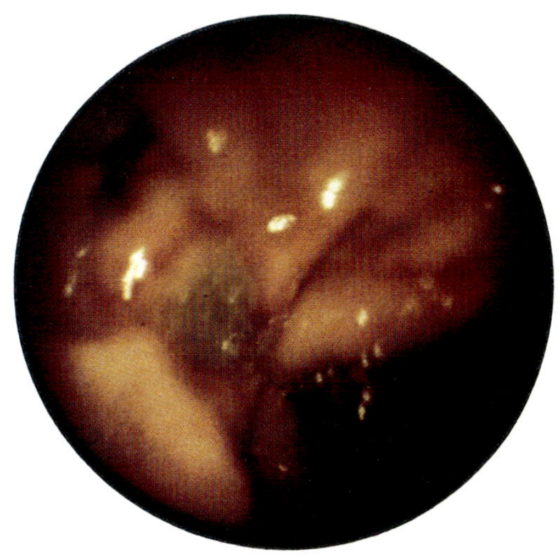

FIG. 11-8 **Ulcer** at pylorus/duodenal junction.

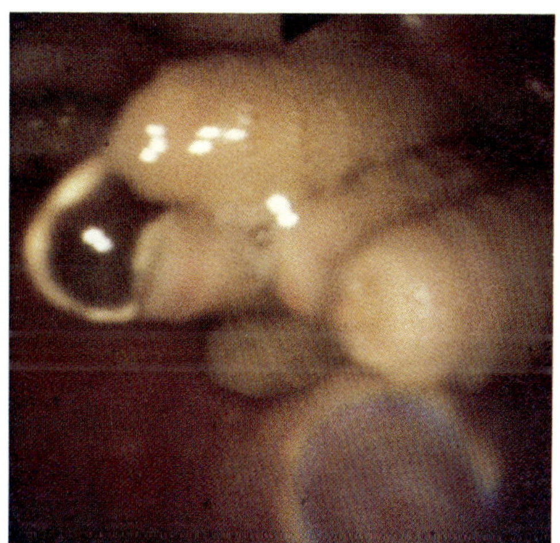

FIG. 11-9 *Gasterophilus nasalis* in duodenum.

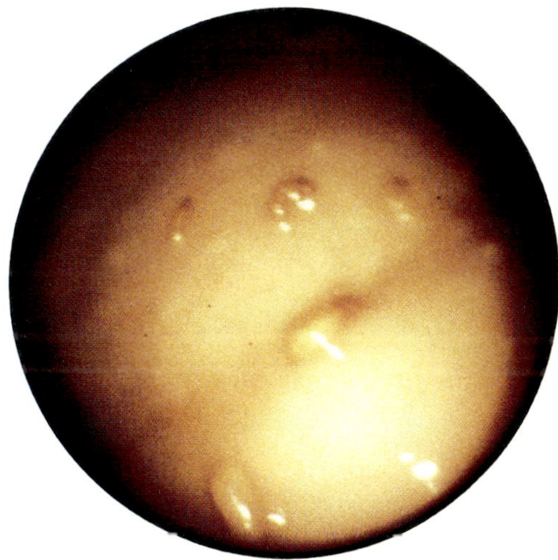

FIG. 11-10 **Duodenal nodules** associated with *Gasterophilus* spp.

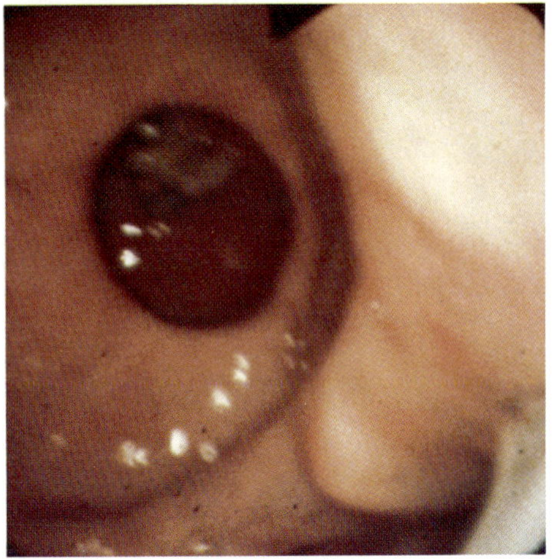

FIG. 11-11 *Gasterophilus* spp. duodenum observed through pylorus.

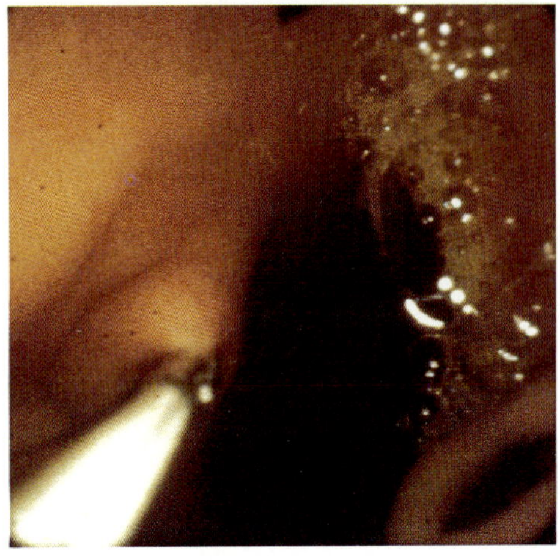

FIG. 11-12 **Duodenal biopsy** opposite the duodenal diverticulum.

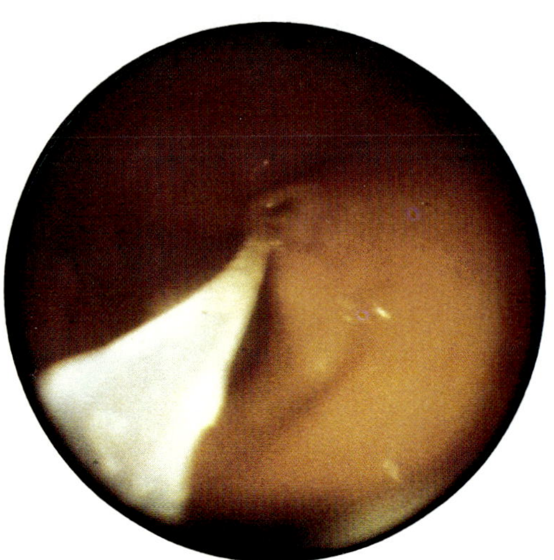

FIG. 11-13 **Aspiration tube** in bile duct.

Chapter 12

Urinary tract

KENNETH E. SULLINS

Genitourinary endoscopy has become the standard of practice for elucidation of lesions that produce dysuria, hematuria, anuria, pyuria, or hemospermia. Indirect evidence of renal or ureteral disease can be obtained by observation or by collection of urine from the specific proximal location. In addition to its use in diagnosis, the endoscope serves as a means to reach lesions with retrieval, electrosurgical, or laser instrumentation. If desired, medication can also be placed directly onto previously diagnosed lesions through the endoscopic channel.

TECHNIQUE OF EXAMINATION

Endoscopy of the equine urinary tract is a simple, atraumatic procedure that can be performed in the standing patient. Endoscopes less than 1 cm in diameter allow free access to the urethrae of males and females. The female urethra is more compliant than that of the male. Smaller diameter endoscopes are generally more flexible, allow more a complete examination, and are necessary to enter the urethra of most male horses. The endoscope should be ≥ 100 cm long to adequately examine the bladder of the adult male horse. The only substantial difference between endoscopy of the genitourinary tract and more common sites, such as the upper airway, is the need for asepsis. Sterilization of the endoscope is covered in Chapter 1.

For safety of personnel, horses, and equipment, restraining the patient in a set of stocks is recommended. Sedating the patient expedites the procedure, helps to prevent breaks in aseptic technique, and is required for access to the male genitourinary tract. Xylazine (0.22 to 0.66 mg/kg, IV) alone or combined with butorphanol (0.02 mg/kg, IV) provides sufficient restraint in most cases. Acepromazine (0.02 mg/kg, IV) in addition to the above IV sedation will improve penile extension if necessary. Overdosage with acepromazine should be avoided because of the risk of penile paralysis. Epidural anesthesia is helpful when mares strain due to severe vaginal or perineal irritation. Since mucus contained in equine urine usually precludes submerged endoscopy, the bladder should be relatively empty. Distension of the urethra and bladder with air is required for adequate visualization. Water inflation will allow visualization of the male urethra, but is more cumbersome. The only advantage of water distention is that it allows control of hemorrhage when necessary.

Mares should have the tail wrapped and tied to their side with a line around the neck. The caudal gluteal, ischial, and perineal regions should be washed with a nonirritating scrub and rinsed completely. Manual and visual examination of the internal vault before endoscopy will familiarize the clinician with the conditions to expect. The endoscope is aseptically introduced into the vulva. The most efficient method of entering the urethra is to locate the urethral orifice with a finger on the free hand and pass the endoscope beneath it. When the anatomy is abnormal, the vulvar and vaginal vault can be inspected by sealing the labia and by using the endoscope to inflate the vault with air.

In the normal mare, the urethra is quite short, and the endoscope encounters the bladder sphincter within 1 to 2 cm of the external urethral orifice. Fortunately, few conditions require extensive evaluation of the female urethra because it is difficult to examine. Once in the bladder, the free hand seals the urethra around the endoscope to allow distention of the bladder with air pumped through the endoscope. Orientation is gained by reference to the residual urine pool in the ventral aspect of the bladder.

Males require sedation to extend the penis enough to grasp for cleansing and insertion of the endoscope (Fig. 12-1). A sterile, water-soluble lubricant should be applied to the endoscope (away from the lens). An assistant wears sterile gloves to handle the penis and endoscope. The examiner handles the eyepiece and controls of the endoscope and need not wear gloves unless sterile catheters or biopsy instruments are to be passed down the channel. Urethral distention is required for examination and is attained by the assistant sealing the urethra around the endoscope. Periodic release of pressure or aspiration with the suction apparatus on the endoscope is

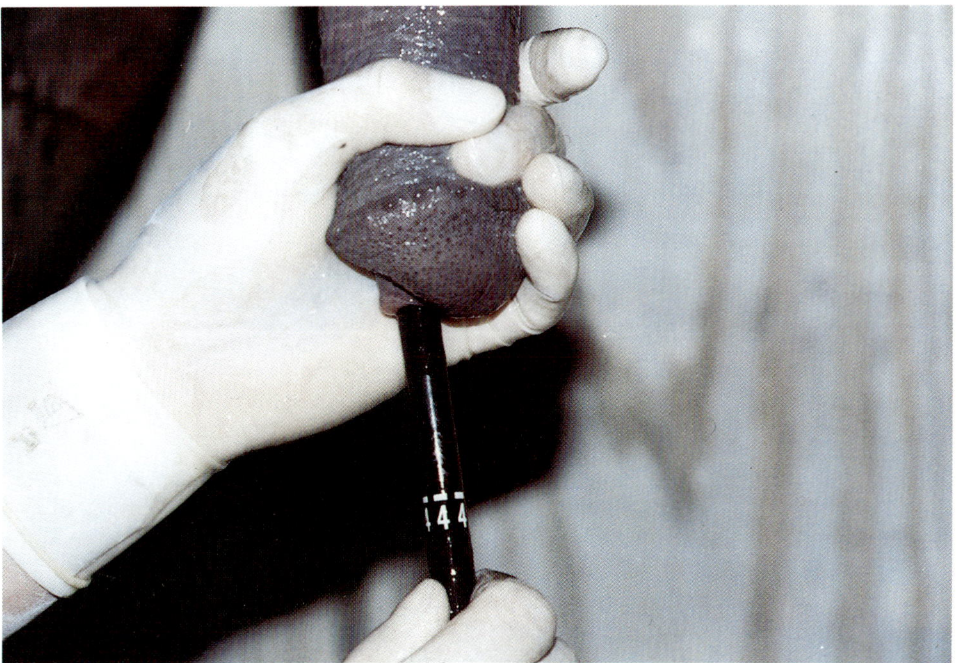

FIG. 12-1   **Manipulation of the penis with the endoscope inserted.**

necessary to prevent overdistention of the bladder. The horse will periodically urinate fluid and air around the endoscope when pressure accumulates.

NORMAL ENDOSCOPIC ANATOMY

Male urethra

The male urethral mucosa is pale and contains numerous longitudinal folds similar to the esophagus (Fig. 12-2). Distention with fluid or air is necessary to see all the mucosal surface. As distention increases, the pale mucosa becomes thinned, revealing the blood in the surrounding cavernous tissue, which appears as multiple dark plaques (Fig. 12-3). These disappear with reduction in pressure and are normal. Detailed examination of the urethra should be performed during the first pass into the bladder because irritation soon causes hyperemia, which complicates interpretation of the findings. No difference is observed between the distal to proximal urethral mucosa until the endoscope has turned around the ischial arch to the pelvic urethra.

Two rows of bulbourethral gland ducts are located mid-dorsally in the distal (caudal) pelvic urethra (Fig. 12-4). Parallel and bilaterally abaxial to those are single rows of lateral urethral glands (Fig. 12-5). In the dorsal urethral wall approximately 3 cm proximal

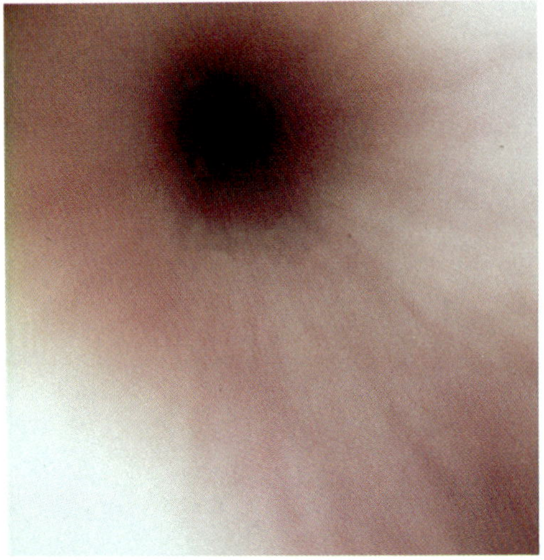

FIG. 12-2   Normal male urethra.
Note the longitudinal folds and
underlying cavernous tissue.

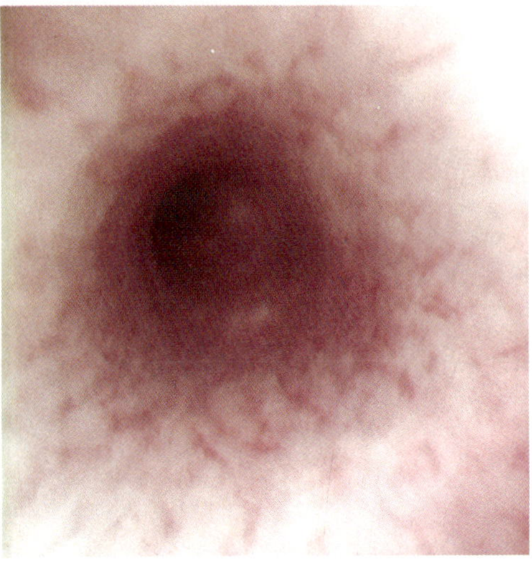

FIG. 12-3   Dark plaques of blood
within the cavernous tissue revealed by
distention of the penile urethra.

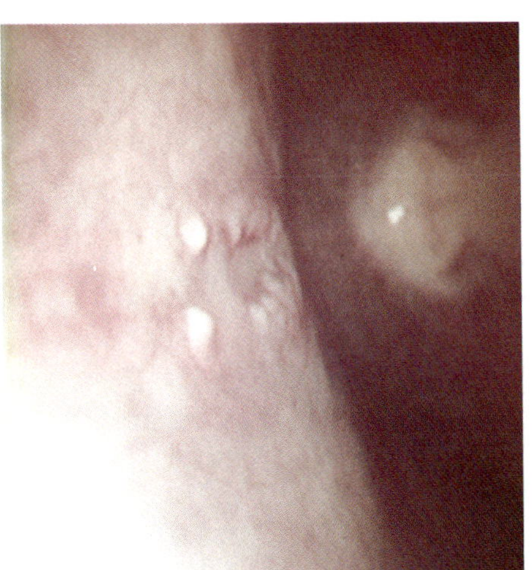

**FIG. 12-4   Two rows of
bulbourethral gland ducts** on dorsal
wall of pelvic urethra. Colliculus
seminalis is in the background.

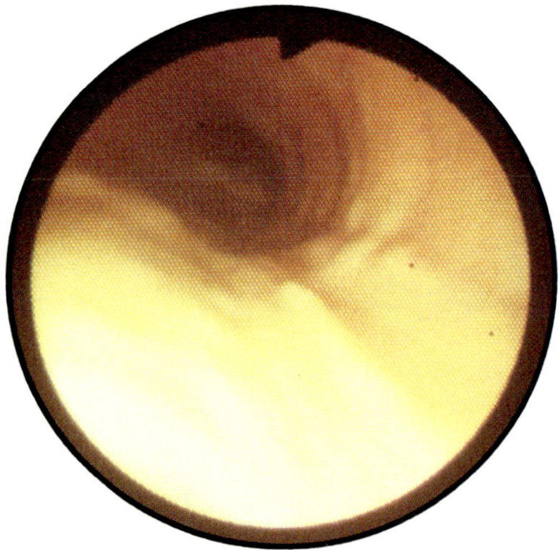

FIG. 12-5   Caudal pelvic urethra
showing ducts of bulbourethral glands
and lateral urethral glands. The
colliculus seminalis is in the left
background (cranial).

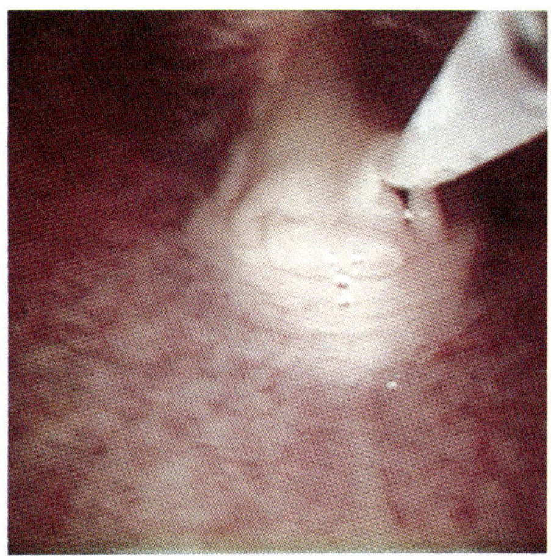

FIG. 12-6 Catheterization of left
ejaculatory duct.

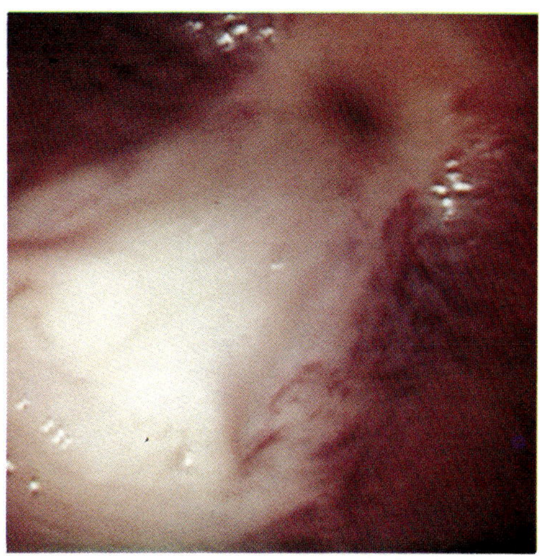

FIG. 12-7 Colliculus seminalis
immediately caudal to urethral sphincter.

(cranial) to these duct orifices are the ejaculatory ducts beside the colliculus seminalis (Fig. 12-6). The circumferential urethral sphincter lies immediately cranial to the colliculus seminalis (Fig. 12-7). Slight resistance may be encountered in passing the endoscope into the bladder. Distention of the urethra will visibly dilate the sphincter and facilitate passage.

Urinary bladder

The cystic mucosa is "soft pink" but becomes darker, and the intramural vasculature becomes more evident when distended with air. Often, a urachal remnant is present as a small (≤1 cm) diverticulum in the bladder wall, cranial to the pool of urine (Figs. 12-8 and 12-9). While keeping the pool ventral, the endoscope is retracted to the neck of the bladder at the cranial margin of the sphincter for observation of the ureteral orifices (Fig. 12-10). These appear abaxially symmetric as slightly oblique paired slits on the dorsal wall of the neck of the bladder. If observed for several seconds to a few minutes, pulsatile urine flow can be seen entering the bladder (Fig. 12-11). The contractile wave moving the fluid down the ureteric column can be observed for its entire intramural length. Function of each ureter should be visually confirmed no matter where the ureter may be located (particularly if nephrectomy or ureteral surgery is contemplated). Particularly, when the ureters are in abnormal locations, observation of urine is facilitated by intravenous administration of fluorescein sodium (6.6 mg/kg) (Fig. 12-12). Ultraviolet filters are available for endoscopic light but are often not necessary to see the yellow-green urine. The urine becomes stained within 5

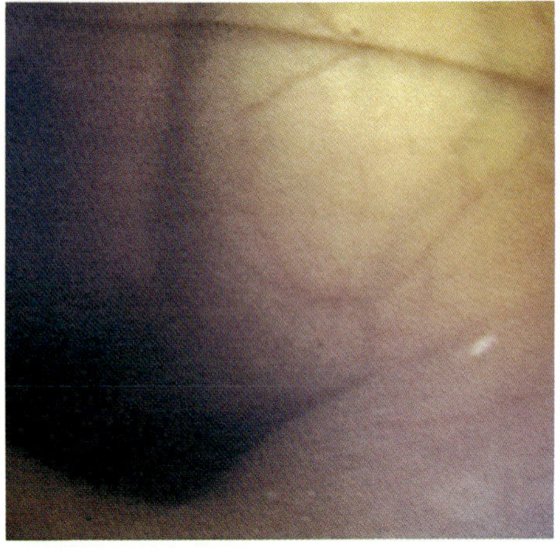

FIG. 12-8 **Remnant of the urachus** in the apex of the bladder viewed under a pool of urine in the floor of the bladder.

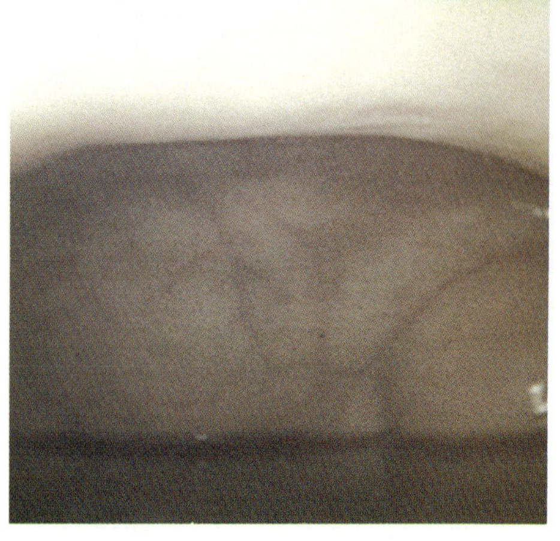

FIG. 12-9 **Apex of the bladder** viewed above a pool of urine in the bladder floor.

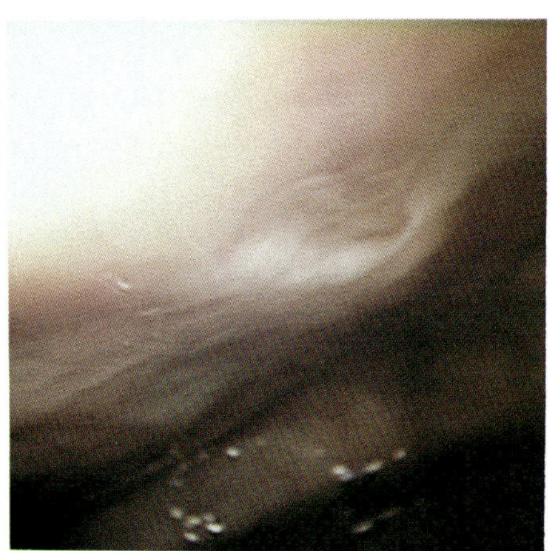

FIG. 12-10 **A normal ureteral orifice.**

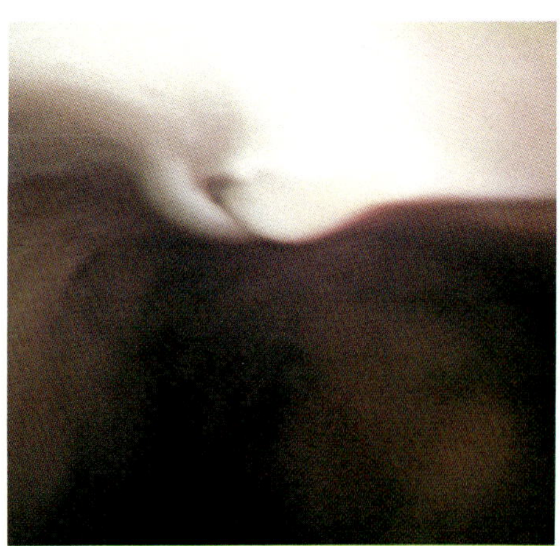

FIG. 12-11 **A normal ureteral orifice** with normal urine passing into the bladder.

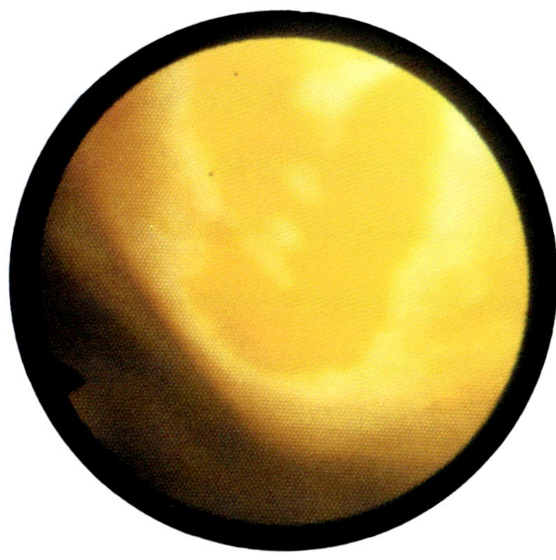

FIG. 12-12   Fluorescein-stained urine entering bladder through ureteral orifice. This procedure helps locate ureters in abnormal locations.

(From Sullins KE and Traub-Dargatz, JL: Endoscopic anatomy of the equine urinary tract, Comp Cont Ed 6(11):S663, 1984.)

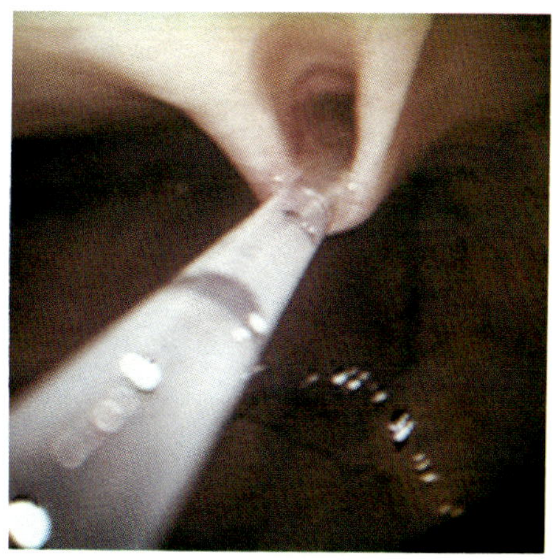

FIG. 12-13   Polyethylene tubing has been placed in the ureter.

minutes of administration. If desired, ureters can be catheterized with sterile polyethylene tubing (PE-205), with a flame-polished end passed through the biopsy channel of the endoscope (Fig. 12-13).

SELECTED ABNORMALITIES

Inflamed urethral mucous membranes are hyperemic and may or may not have fibrinonecrotic debris adherent to the surface or free in the lumen (Fig. 12-14). Surface ulceration may be present, and bleeding granulation tissue may fill the defects. The exudate will be purulent but may be diluted by varying amounts of urine or mucus. The presenting complaint will often be repeated, unsuccessful attempts to urinate or diminished urination. Aside from infection or primary injury (e.g., stallion rings, calculi, kick wounds), necrosis or erosion of tumors can produce similar signs. Bladder inflammation is usually much less impressive than when observed in the urethra (Fig. 12-15), but urinary calculi are easily located (Fig. 12-16).

Another common complaint is hematuria or hemospermia. Blood may appear when emitted or simply be discovered dried on the hindlimbs of stallions or geldings. Blood in the urine often clears during early micturition if it is urethral in origin. If it persists during the entire micturition or appears at the end, the bladder or

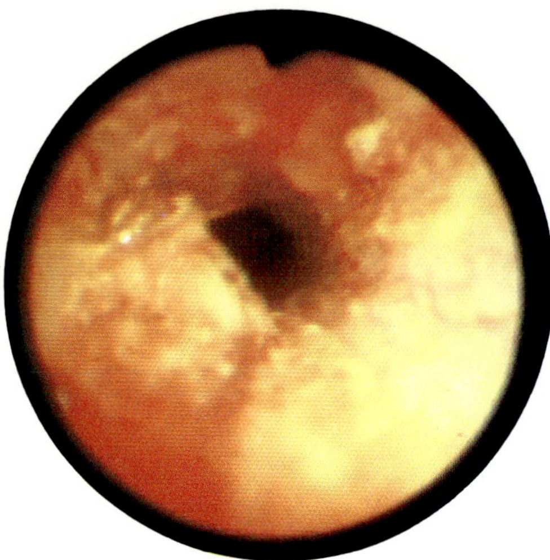

FIG. 12-14   Bacterial urethritis with fibrinous exudate.

(Courtesy Dr NT Messer, IV.)

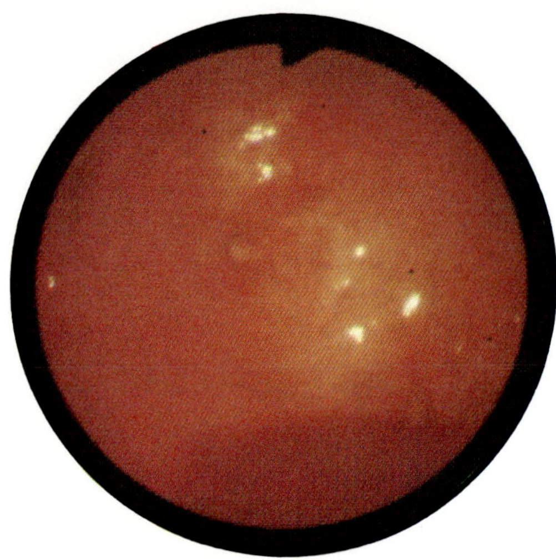

FIG. 12-15   Inflamed mucosa of bladder with cystitis. Small amount of urine is present on the floor.

(From Sullins KE and Traub-Dargatz JL: Comp Cont Ed 6(11):S663, 1984.)

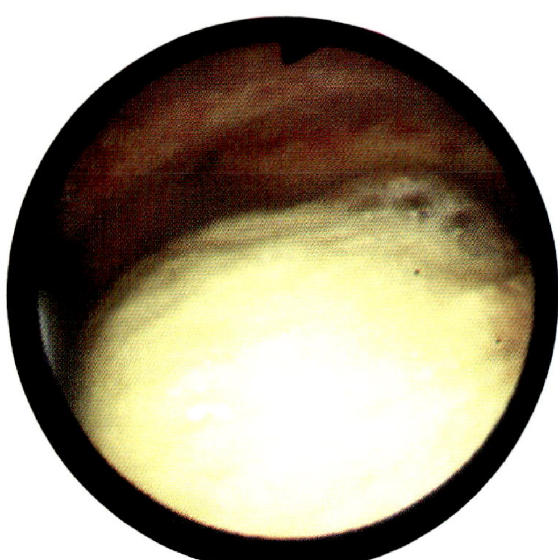

FIG. 12-16   Calculus in the bladder.

(From Sullins KE and Traub-Dargatz JL: Comp Cont Ed 6(11):S663, 1984.)

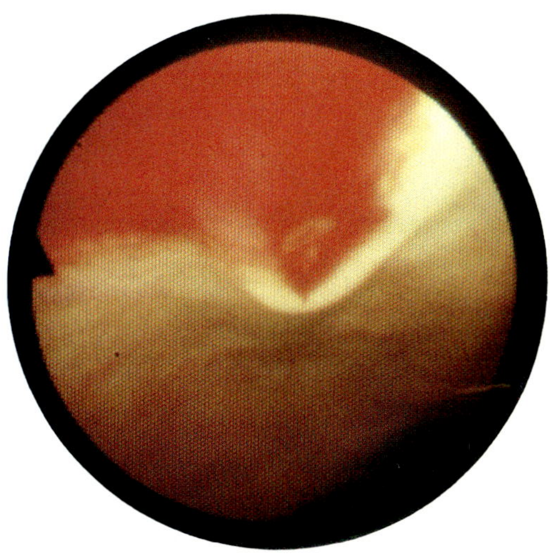

FIG. 12-17 Hemorrhagic urine entering bladder from unilaterally affected kidney.

(From Sullins KE and Traub-Dargatz JL: Comp Cont Ed 6(11):S663, 1984.)

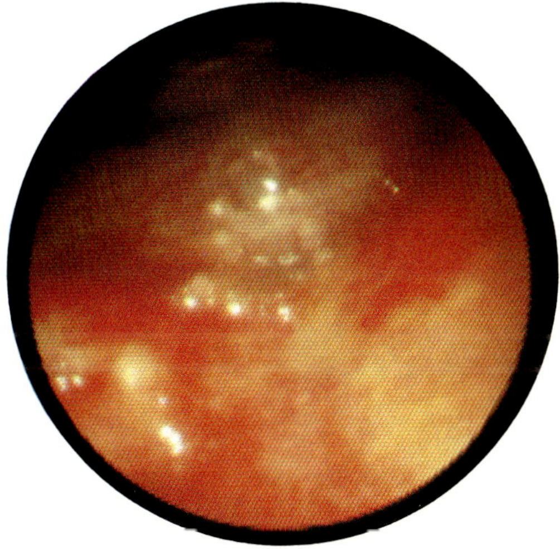

FIG. 12-18 Varicosity in the pelvic urethra. The colliculus seminalis is in the background.

(From Sullins KE and Traub-Dargatz JL: Comp Cont Ed 6(11):S663, 1984.)

kidneys should be suspected (Fig. 12-17). However, some urethral hemorrhage occurs only during the muscular contraction at the end of urination. Hemospermia usually results from lesions that exacerbate with increased cavernous pressure. Fissures in the urethral membrane may go undetected unless the stallion is examined during detumescence. Other lesions may appear as permanent varicosities (Fig. 12-18) or ulcerations, which are most commonly found in the pelvic urethra adjacent to the colliculus seminalis. A combination of these signs can appear if inflammation accompanies or instigates the corpus cavernosum hemorrhage.

Table 12-1 lists common diseases or abnormalities encountered during endoscopic examination.

TABLE 12-1 Common diseases or abnormalities encountered during endoscopic examination of the equine genitourinary tract.

STRUCTURE	SEX	COMPLAINT	CONDITION	COMMENTS
Urethra	Male	Dysuria, hemospermia	Urethritis	Inflammation[6,8]
	Male	Hemospermia	Corpus cavernous hemorrhage	Usually a slit or varicosity in pelvic urethra; rarely seen in geldings[4,7,8,10]
	Male	Dysuria, anuria	Urolithiasis	Usually lodge at ischial arch; more common in bladder[1,6,7]
	Male	Dysuria, hematuria, or hemospermia	Neoplasia	Squamous cell carcinoma, melanoma, papilloma, sarcoid[5]
	Male	Dysuria, incontinence	Ectopic ureter	Possible cystitis[5]
Bladder	Either	Dysuria, hematuria, anuria	Urinary calculi	Usually males[2]
		Hematuria	Idiopathic, Renal Disease (Pyelonephritis, PBZ Toxicity)	Observe urine from each ureter (uni- or bilateral); catheterize ureter if necessary
		Dysuria, hematuria	Cystitis	Thick/granulating wall; fibrinonecrotic mucosa[3]
		Dysuria, pyuria, hematuria	Neoplasia	Cystic transitional cell carcinoma, renal cell carcinoma (ureteral hemorrhage)
Ureter	Either	None, pain	Ureterolith	Observe lack of ureteral urine flow; may reach with catheter or basket[1]
Vagina/ Vulva	Mare	Incontinence	Ectopic ureter	Observe urine flow or catheterize and radiograph; observed in vaginal floor or cervix[5]

REFERENCES

1. DeBowes RM: Obstructive urinary tract disease. In Robinson NE, editor: Current therapy in equine medicine, ed 2, Philadelphia, 1987, WB Saunders Co.
2. DeBowes RM, Nyrop KA, and Boulton CH: Cystic calculi in the horse, Comp Cont Ed 6(5):S268, 1984.
3. Hodgson DR: Cystitis and pyelonephritis. In Robinson NE, editor: Current therapy in equine medicine, ed 2, Philadelphia, 1987, WB Saunders Co.
4. Hurtgen JP: Stallion genital abnormalities. In Robinson NE, editor: Current therapy in equine medicine, ed 2, Philadelphia, 1987, WB Saunders Co.
5. Modransky P: Neoplastic and anomalous conditions of the urinary tract. In Robinson NE, editor: Current therapy in equine medicine, ed 2, Philadelphia, 1987, WB Saunders Co.
6. Robertson JT: Conditions of the urethra. In Robinson NE, editor: Current therapy in equine medicine, ed 2, Philadelphia, 1987, WB Saunders Co.
7. Sullins KE and Traub-Dargatz JL: Endoscopic anatomy of the equine urinary tract, Comp Cont Ed 6(11):S663, 1984.
8. Sullins KE et al: Treatment of hemospermia in stallions: A discussion of 18 cases, Comp Cont Ed, 10(12):1396, 1988.
9. Traub JL: Intraabdominal neoplasia as a cause of chronic weight loss in the horse, Comp Cont Ed 5(10):S526, 1983.
10. Voss JL and Wottoway JL: Hemospermia, Proc 18th Ann Conv Am Assoc Equine Pract 18:103-110, 1972.

Chapter 13

Mare's Genital Tract

CARLA L. CARLETON AND WALTER R. THRELFALL

Endoscopy of the mare's genital tract has proved beneficial in the assessment of fertility when the more common methods have been inadequate. Initially, a thorough breeding, foaling, and disease history should be taken. A complete breeding soundness examination, consisting of transrectal palpation, vaginal examination, uterine culture, cytology, endometrial biopsy, and ultrasonography should be performed when mare fertility is in question. The next diagnostic procedure in the abnormal or otherwise apparently normal mare suffering from chronic infertility would be endoscopy. In mares with palpable defects, discharges, or unusual ultrasonographic examinations, the endoscope can aid in diagnosis, treatment, and prognosis.

The majority of veterinary practices own only one endoscope, which may be used primarily for respiratory tract endoscopic examinations. Keeping this in mind, and remembering that many upper respiratory tract microorganisms are also associated with infertility in the mare—especially streptococci—it is essential that the endoscope be sterilized before its introduction into the genital tract.

EQUIPMENT

The equipment suitable for examination of the mare's reproductive tract is a flexible fiberscope (gastroscope or colonoscope), no less than 1 m long (preferably 180 mm) and 12 to 14 mm in diameter, with a cold light source and an anterior viewing field. Essential options or accessories are jet flushing of the viewing window, biopsy capability, suction, photo and/or video for medical records, air pump, and numerous snares. The endoscope must be immersible for sterilization.[4,6,13,17]

Additional optional equipment is currently available in human medicine and may eventually gain veterinary application. Examples are the laser, diathermy shock wave generators and hydraulic devices for use in endoscopic surgery.[5,8,14]

EQUIPMENT PREPARATION

A common method of equipment disinfection is by submerging the flexible portion of the endoscope in a glutaraldehyde-based solution[2,3] or in an iodine solution followed by an alcohol rinse.[6,12,15] Recommended contact time with glutaraldehyde solution is 10 minutes; longer times may cause equipment damage. Older equipment may not be suitable for submersion because of possible gasket damage.[7] Care must be taken to include disinfection of the biopsy channel by drawing the glutaraldehyde or iodine solution into the full length of the channel. Likewise, any accessories that will be used during the examination, such as the biopsy instrument and water bottle, also need to be sterilized.

Because glutaraldehyde solutions are extremely irritating, it is essential that all traces of the chemical be rinsed from the endoscope with sterile distilled water[2] before its introduction into the mare's genital tract. Distilled water is preferred for the equipment rinse to minimize crystallization of salts in the equipment channels. Care must be taken not to contaminate the equipment during rinsing.

PREPARATION OF THE MARE

The importance of perineal preparation before endoscopy cannot be overemphasized. It is not suitable to perform an endoscopic examination in a barn or stall because of dust, dirt, and the inability to adequately protect the equipment. Because of the possibility of equipment damage and operator injury should the mare drop in the stocks, it is preferable to have a nonrigid, quick-release rear restraint on the stocks. A car seat belt, a chain with a quick-release handle, or a quick-release rope (tied in a figure eight around a cleat) behind the mare is recommended.

The mare's tail should be wrapped and tied to one side to prevent tail hairs and debris from entering the examination field. A mild detergent or diluted iodine solution can be used to wash the perineum, followed by copious cotton and water rinses. This should be repeated until the cotton rinses reveal no visible contamination. Our wash routine begins on the midline, including the rectal sphincter and vulvar lips, and extends below the region of the clitoris, with washing continuing laterally 10 to 15 cm to both sides. To avoid repeated midline contact with a piece of cotton, discard the cotton once the midline and one side have been cleansed, continuing with another piece of cotton on the midline and laterally, and so on.

Stretching of the circular muscles of the myometrium and the associated discomfort necessitate tranquilizing the mare before an endoscopic examination. Our regimen is to use xylazine (.66 mg/kg) with acepromazine maleate (.044 mg/kg) IV. Our preference for xylazine over butorphanol is based on xylazine's greater analgesia with regard to visceral pain.[9]

TECHNIQUE AND PERSONNEL

The veterinarian lifts the control end of the flexible portion from the glutaraldehyde solution. The assistant, wearing a sterile plastic sleeve on one hand and a sterile glove on the opposite hand, grasps the endoscope. The distal tip of the flexible portion is held in the sleeved hand while the gloved hand grasps the flexible portion at mid-shaft. The assistant holds the scope at an angle, at arms length, while sterile water is poured from the proximal to the distal end, with repeated flushings. The entire flexible portion is rinsed with 1500 to 2000 ml of sterile water. Care must be taken also to rinse the distal tip of the scope by lifting it up and flushing it thoroughly. In addition, the biopsy channel should be flushed liberally with 150 to 200 ml sterile water. The presterilized flush reservoir of the unit should be filled with sterile saline for use during the procedure.

A veterinarian will require at least one assistant to perform an endoscopic examination of the genital tract. The veterinarian visually examines the lumen as the assistant advances and withdraws the endoscope as instructed. Introduction of the scope into the mare's genital tract is facilitated by placing a sterile lubricant on the back of the assistant's gloved hand. Avoid placing lubricant in one's palm, which could result in the viewing lens becoming smeared with lubricant, thus obscuring the view.

EXAMINATION TECHNIQUE AND STRUCTURE
IDENTIFICATION WITHIN THE MARE

As the endoscope is carried through the vulval lips, one may begin to observe the color of the vestibular and vaginal mucosa and the presence and nature of any discharge or abnormal structures. Endoscopy of the vagina can confirm the presence of urine, inflammation, varicosities, or polyps, and possibly the origin of discharges which have been noted at the vulval lips. Feces in the vagina may indicate either poor vulval conformation (and the necessity of a Caslicks or Pourets surgery to correct it) or the presence of a rectovaginal fistula.

The vaginal vault in the normal mare, before the introduction of air, is not hyperemic. Depending on the stage of the cycle, the mucosa may appear more (estrus) or less moist (diestrus). The color is usually a pale pink (Fig. 13-1). As the vaginal examination always follows a transrectal palpation of the genital tract, the degree of cervical relaxation will already have been determined.

The appearance of the diestrual cervix during the vaginal portion of the endoscopic examination will be closed and residing approximately in the center of the cranial vaginal vault (Fig. 13-2). As the cervix relaxes to varying degrees during estrus, it will begin to flatten and drop toward the floor of the vagina. Unless there is an abnormal condition, such as urine pooling, cervicitis (Fig. 13-3), or severe endometritis, there should be no apparent discharge or fluid noted. Unlike the cow, the mare does not discharge large amounts of mucus when in estrus. Adhesions—a reflection of vaginal irritation (which may follow uterine infusion of irritating solutions or treatments inappropriate for the mare), inflammation or infection—may be evident in the vagina. Damage to the cervix and vaginal vault also may be the result of a dystocia, especially those instances when assistance was given prior to adequate cervical relaxation (Fig. 13-4).

As with other uterine procedures in the mare, the index finger is first introduced fully through the cervix. All mare cervices are not perfectly linear, and placement of the index finger through the entire length of the cervical lumen eases the passage of the endoscope. A closed or partially relaxed cervix maintains contact with the endoscope as it passes through the cervical lumen, thus precluding viewing the walls of the cervix.

As the endoscope reaches the internal cervical os, the endometrial folds are the first structures to come into view. If the operator chooses the standard procedure of dilating the lumen as the endoscope is advanced, the endoscope can be guided gently forward into the uterine body and horns. The endometrium can be viewed as the endoscope is introduced to the tip of the uterine horn.

The uterine lumen is a potential space. To examine it, one must dilate the lumen with either fluid or gas.[1,10,11,17] There are reports that favor extreme dilation of the uterus before the introduction of the endoscope.[16] This may preclude identification of fluid or adhesions before they are distorted.

The endometrium is very sensitive and becomes rapidly hyperemic with distension, whether by fluid or air. By dilating the uterus with air, saline, or sterile water as the scope makes its initial pass

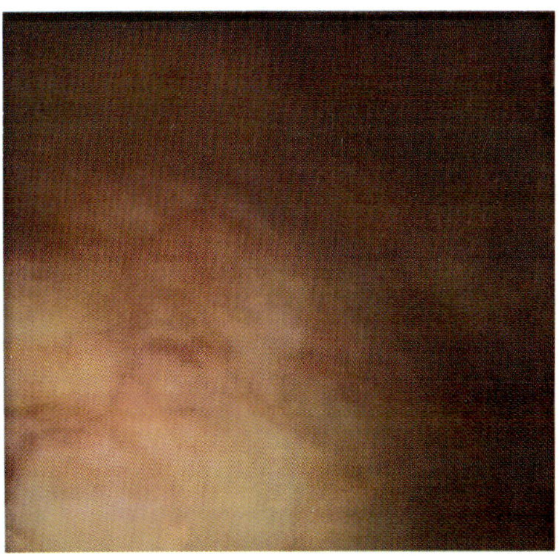

FIG. 13-1 Hyperemic vaginal mucosa induced by pneumovagina.

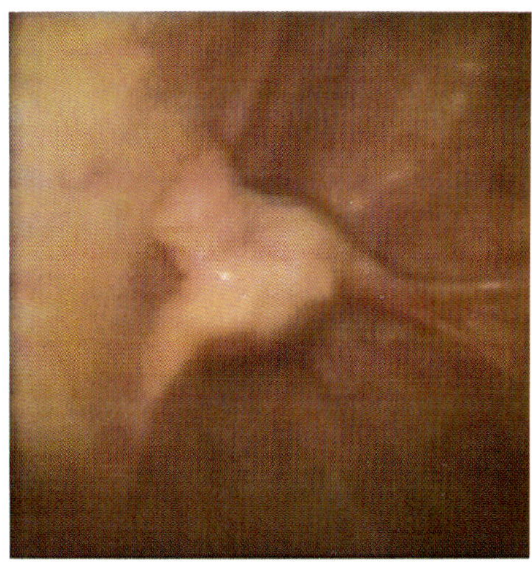

FIG. 13-2 Vaginal endoscopy. Normal external cervical os, closed.

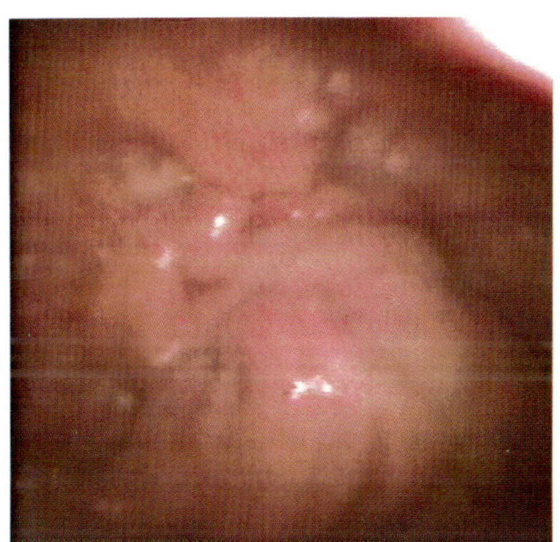

FIG. 13-3 The external cervical os. The hyperemia was secondary to poor vulvar conformation and pneumovagina.

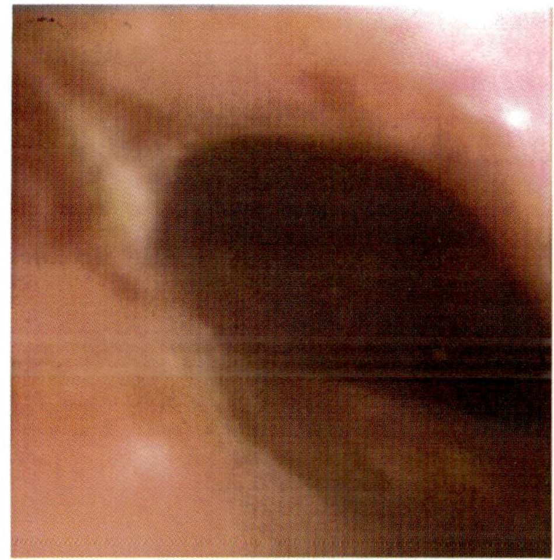

FIG. 13-4 Cervical ulcerations evident 12 days postfoaling. Although the mare was in estrus, the cervix was not merely relaxed but incompetent.

into the lumen, the endometrial folds can be examined as well as any gross abnormalities, if present. Physiological solutions, such as saline, would induce a lesser inflammatory response than hypotonic solutions, such as sterile water.

The endometrial folds are normally pale pink, shiny, and appear as longitudinal folds (Fig. 13-5) reaching from the internal cervical os to the tips of the uterine horns. They number from 12 to 15 in the mare. The character of the normal endometrium and folds is primarily a reflection of the season and stage of the cycle. During the physiologic breeding season (cycling), the endometrial folds should be palpable and visible by endoscopic examination. During estrus the folds are edematous, while in diestrus they appear less prominent and paler.

By observing the lumen as it is filled, one is permitted the opportunity to see the folds first as they completely occupy the luminal potential space (Fig. 13-5). As the endoscope is advanced and the lumen expanded, the folds will appear less prominent (Figs. 13-6–13-9). At this point transluminal adhesions can be readily detected as they stretch across the lumen. The same is true for endometrial cysts whether broad-based or pedunculated. Fluid present in the lumen can also be observed as the uterus fills. With full dilation the folds appear to compress into the wall (Figs. 13-10, 13-11). The folds of the mare in deep winter anestrus or of one suffering from a chronic pyometra or endomyometritis may be less prominent or absent in the noninflated or partially inflated state. By performing a consistent technique, one becomes more adept at viewing small transluminal adhesions, fluid, exudate, and plaques before they are disrupted by expansion or diluted by the filling solution.

The normal landmark at the cranial end of the uterine body is the bifurcation of the uterine horns (Fig. 13-12). It appears as a frenulum with a lumen to either side. The examining veterinarian stipulates the speed at which the scope is to be advanced and can direct the head into either the left or the right uterine horn.

There are cases in which complete luminal adhesions have formed. In light of this, it is necessary to determine during an endoscopic examination if the entire uterine horn has been traversed. One could surmise from the earlier transrectal examination the approximate length of the genital tract (vagina, cervix, uterine body and horn) and how much of the scope should enter the mare. More objective than that is the identification of the ostium at the uterotubal junction. It protrudes as a tiny bump into the tip of the uterine horn (Figs. 13-11, 13-13). Positive identification of this structure eliminates all uncertainty.

Inflammation, adhesions, cystic structures, and degenerative endometrial changes may affect the appearance of the endometrium.

Text continued on p. 166.

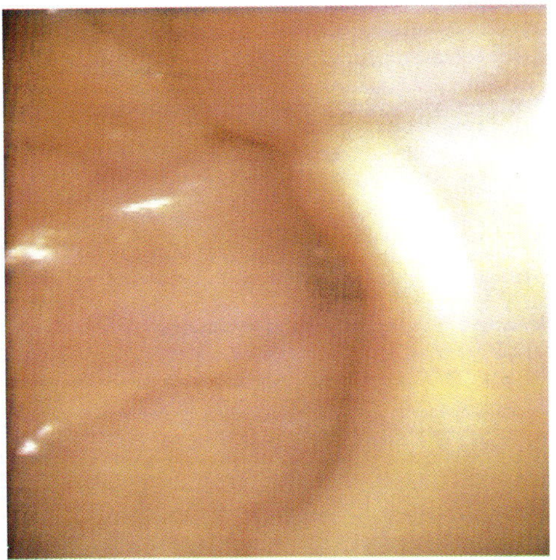

FIG. 13-5 Normal endometrium.
Appearance of the folds prior to fluid
expansion of the lumen.

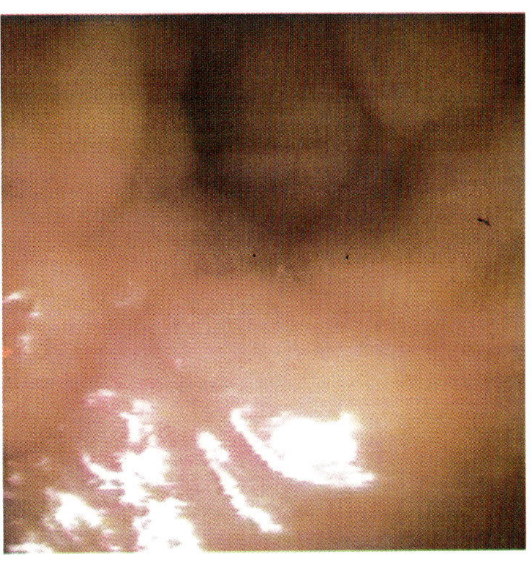

**FIG. 13-6 Normal endometrium:
color and folds.** Luminal dilation is
partial.

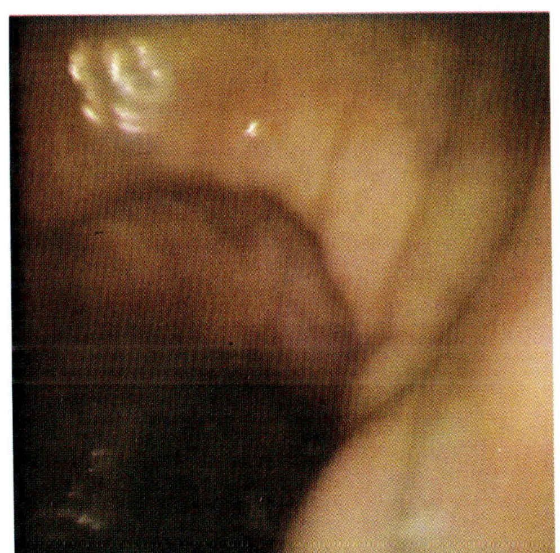

FIG. 13-7 Normal endometrial folds.
Partial luminal distention.

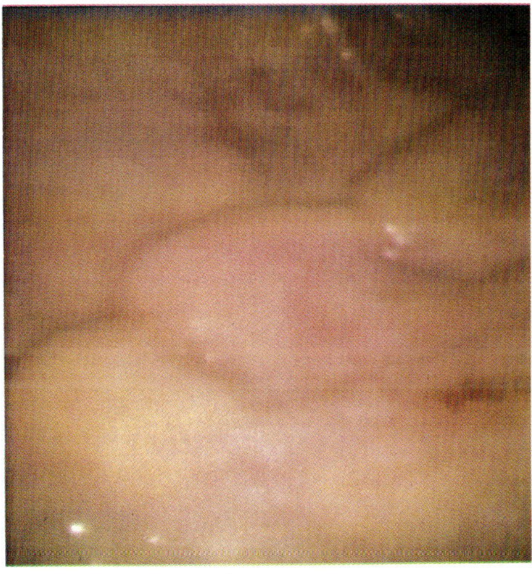

**FIG. 13-8 Normal endometrium and
folds.** Luminal dilation approximately
50%.

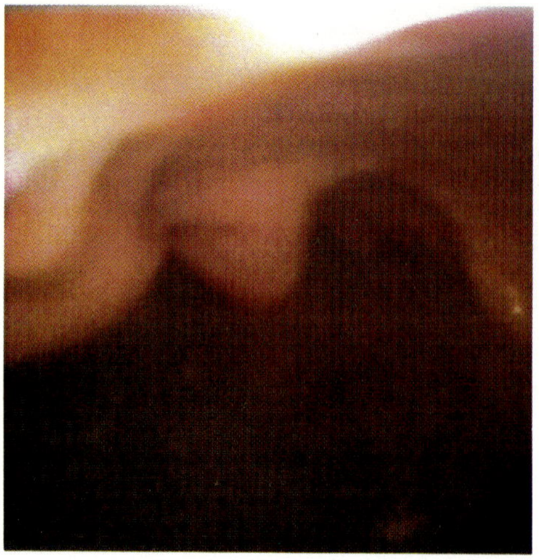

FIG. 13-9   Normal endometrial folds. Expansion of the lumen is almost complete.

FIG. 13-10   Normal endometrium, expansion of lumen ("compression of folds") complete. The endometrium can become hyperemic within a short time. Unless it was noted at the outset, it is likely a result of the procedure.

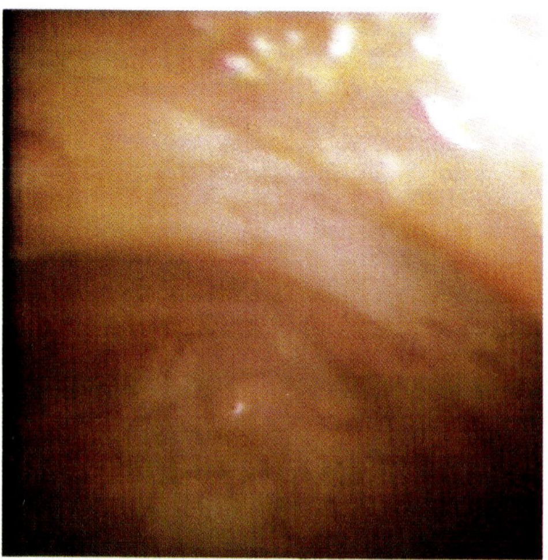

FIG. 13-11   Uterine horn dilation complete. Approaching apical end of uterine horn. Uterotubal ostium is in view.

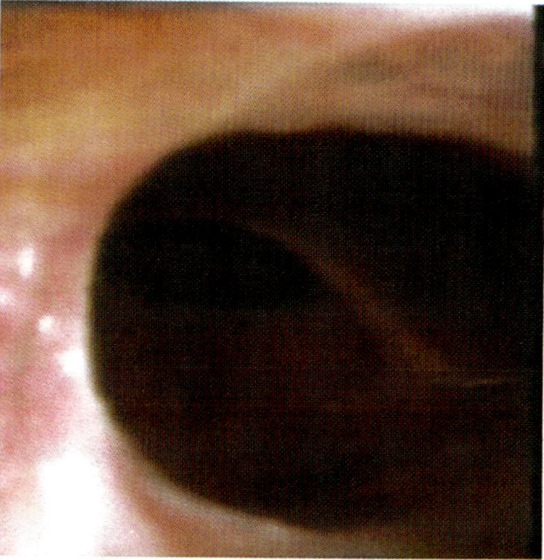

FIG. 13-12 Lumen completely dilated at the level of the uterine body and horns. The bifurcation of the horns appears as a central dividing frenulum.

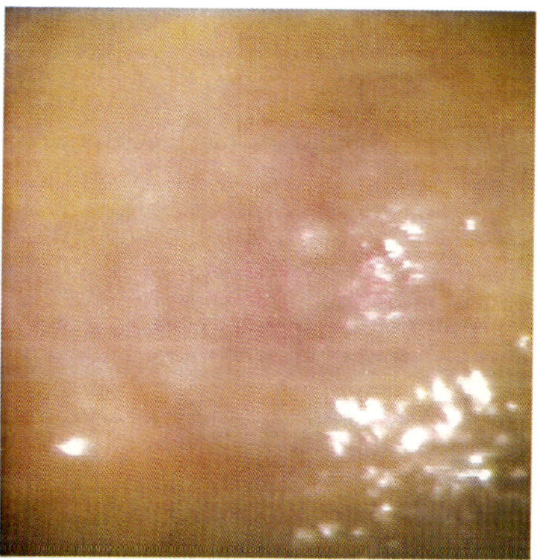

FIG. 13-13 The apical end of the uterine horn at which the ostium (uterotubal junction) can be seen.

Acute or chronic infections, dystocia or obstetrical manipulations, or genital surgery may have been the inciting cause of the abnormalities observed (Table 13-1).

Endometrial cysts are increasingly more common as mares age. While small cysts (10 to 15 mm) may be insignificant (Fig. 13-14) if few in number, some concern exists that larger cysts may have a detrimental effect on the mare's fertility (Figs. 13-15–13-19), perhaps by inhibition of the transuterine migration of the early conceptus. *Candida* sp. infections (Fig. 13-31), in our experience, create large amounts of a viscous fluid within the uterus, in addition to adherent, stringy, endometrial plaques.

Examples of foreign bodies first detected by palpation or ultrasonography and identified by endoscopy are fetal mummy (resolved twin after calcification has occurred), culture swab tip, manure (suggesting severe pneumovagina, incompetent cervix, poor vulval conformation), etc.

Foreign bodies may cause varying degrees of reduced fertility or infertility. The endoscopic findings must be correlated with those of additional investigations (including tissue biopsies and cultures), together with the history and transrectal palpation findings.

Clearly, if an abnormality has been palpated or detected by ultrasonography, then the goal is to determine if it is luminal. If it is, then it is possible to perform biopsy, aspiration, curettage, surgery, etc., to correct the problem. Opaque luminal fluids such as urine, pus, or mucus can present some difficulty in complete visualization of the endometrium. While a saline flush of the uterus prior to an endoscopic exam may cause hyperemia of the endometrium, it may be necessary if the lumen is to be evaluated.

Text continued on p. 172.

TABLE 13-1 Abnormalities of the reproductive tract of the mare which may be seen endoscopically

CONDITION	CLINICAL SIGNS
Vaginitis/vaginal hyperemia (Fig. 13-3)	Often associated with abnormal conformation and pneumovagina; if infected, vaginal discharge may be present.
Cervical lacerations and scars (Fig. 13-4)	Infertility in some cases
Endometrial cysts (Figs. 13-14, 13-19)	Possibly infertile
Endometrial lacerations (Fig. 13-20)	Possibly infertile
Endometrial hyperemia (Fig. 13-21)	Usually none
Purulent endometritis (Figs. 13-22, 13-23)	Infertility; possible vaginal discharge
Uterine luminal adhesions and scarring (Figs. 13-24 to 13-30)	Infertility
Fungal plaque (Fig. 13-31)	Possible infertility and discharge

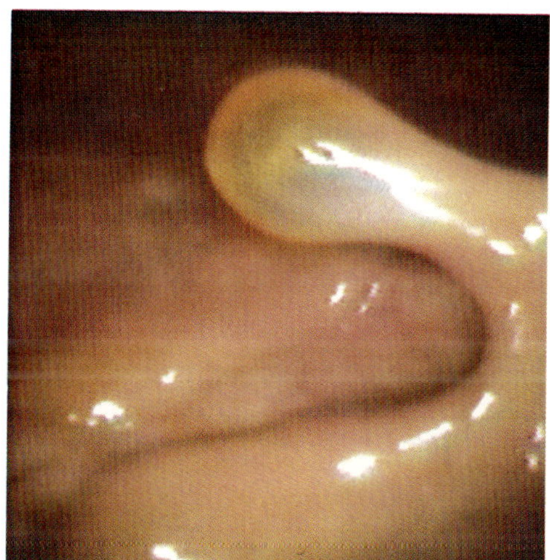

FIG. 13-14 **Pedunculated endometrial cyst,** narrow base and stalk.

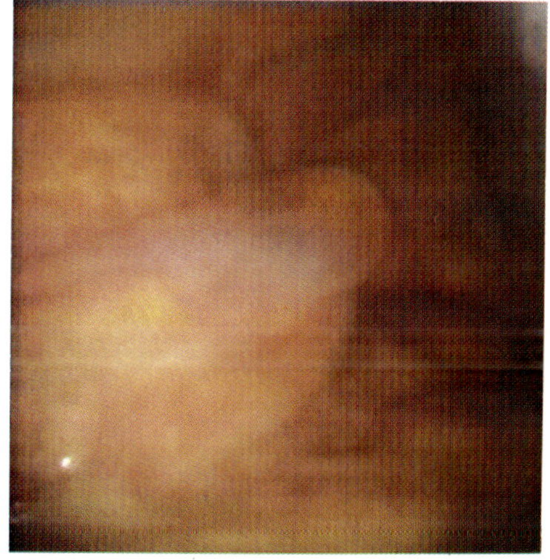

FIG. 13-15 **Pedunculated endometrial cyst,** broader base.

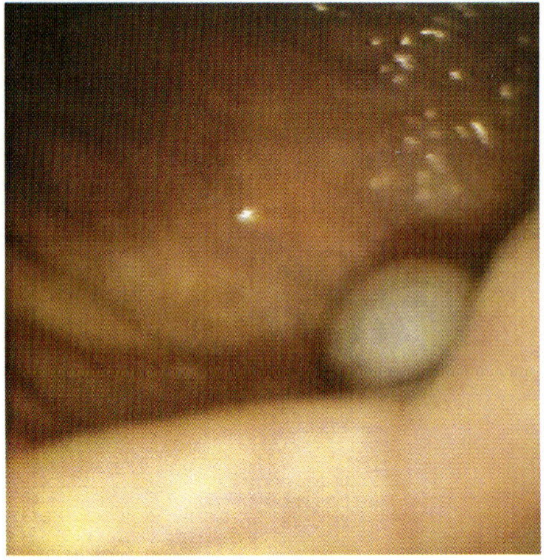

FIG. 13-16   A thin-walled, broad-based endometrial cyst.

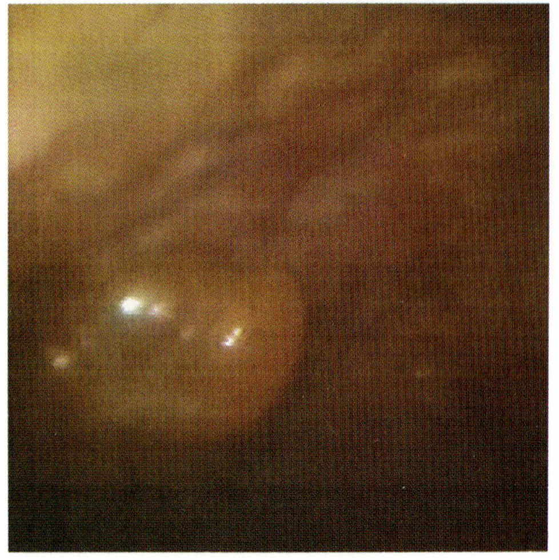

FIG. 13-17   A multilocular, broad-based endometrial cyst.

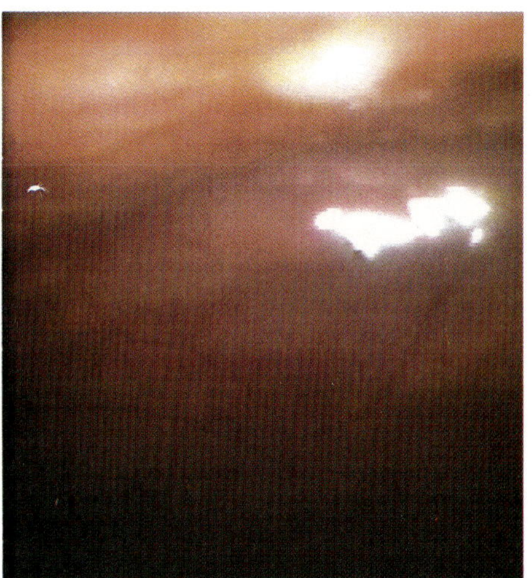

FIG. 13-18   Large uterine cyst. It measured 5.5 cm. The cyst fills the bottom three-quarters of the field of view.

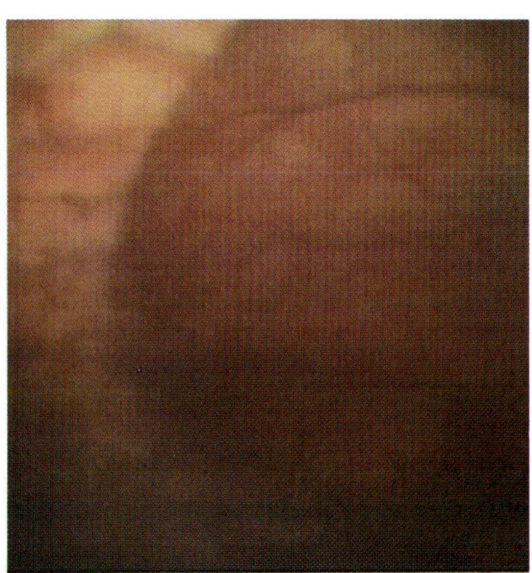

FIG. 13-19   Large spherical endometrial cyst occupying most of the lumen.

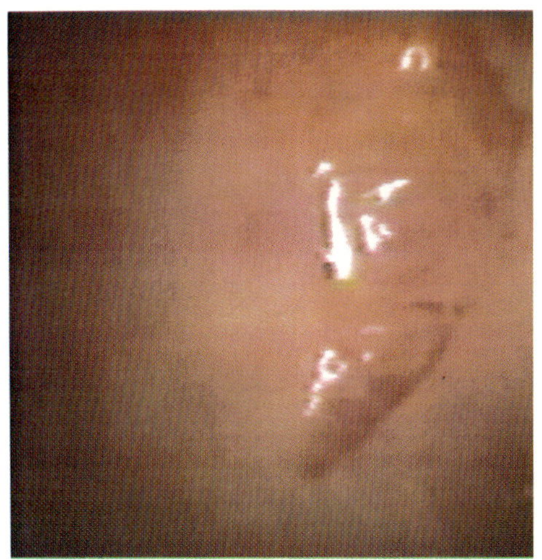

FIG. 13-20 **Laceration of the endometrium.** The mare had been purchased recently. No history available.

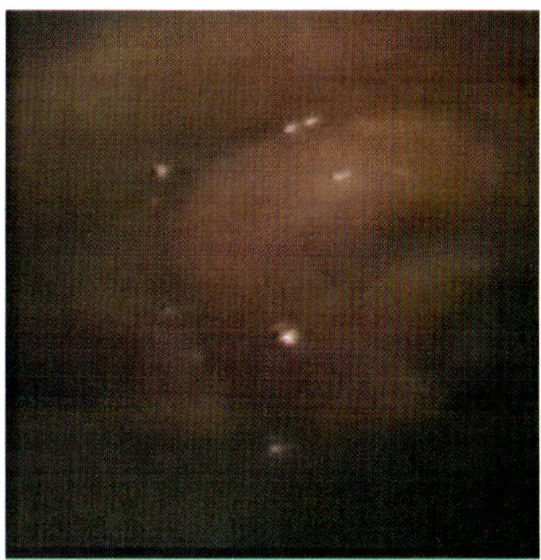

FIG. 13-21 **Hyperemic endometrial folds** before expansion of the uterine lumen.

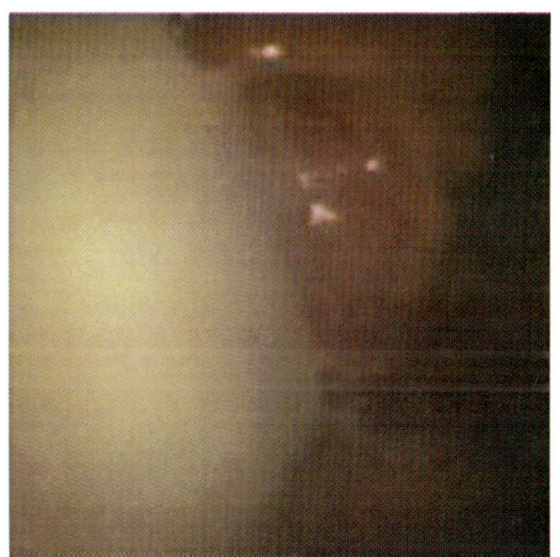

FIG. 13-22 **Translucent purulent fluid** in the lumen. The mare had a positive culture for beta hemolytic streptococcus.

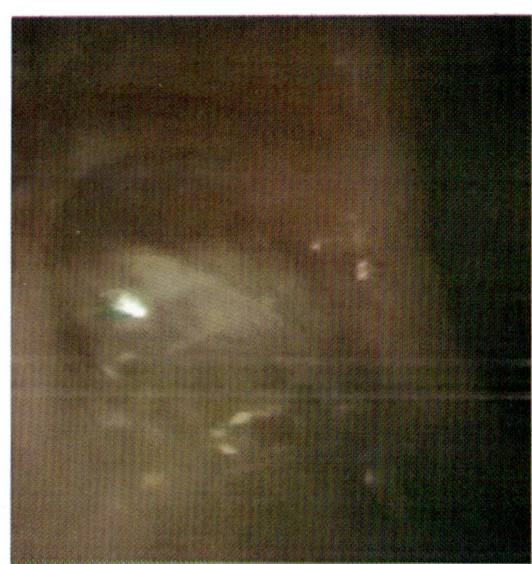

FIG. 13-23 **Less viscous purulent fluid** accumulation in the lumen.

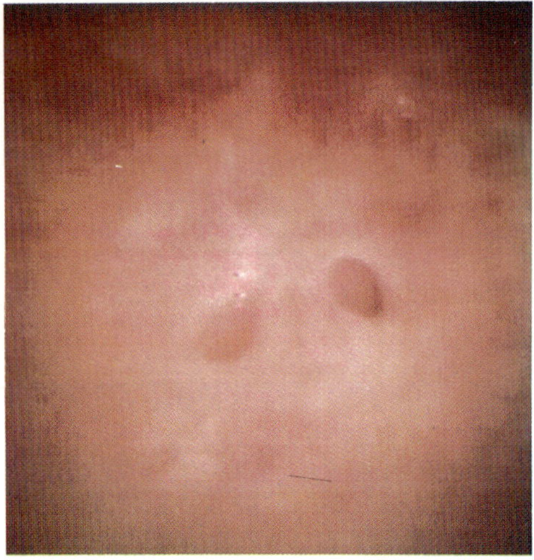

FIG. 13-24 Wall of scar tissue obliterating the uterine lumen. The two small fenestrations are the only remaining communication to the apical portion of the horn.

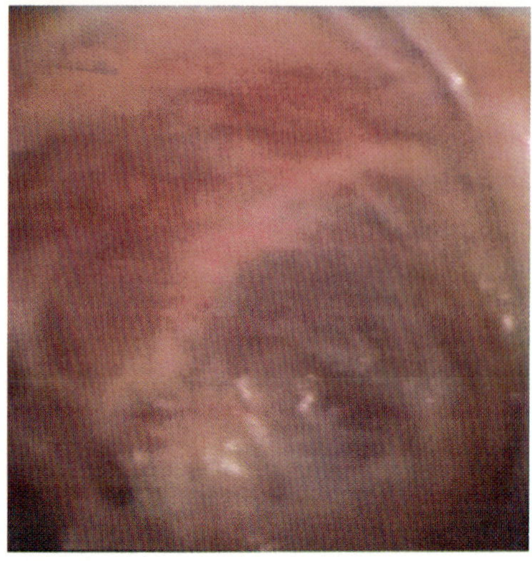

FIG. 13-25   Extensive uterine adhesions. This mare had a positive culture for beta hemolytic streptococcus. In addition to having a history of infertility, the current inflammatory reaction followed treatment of her uterine infection, antibiotic unknown.

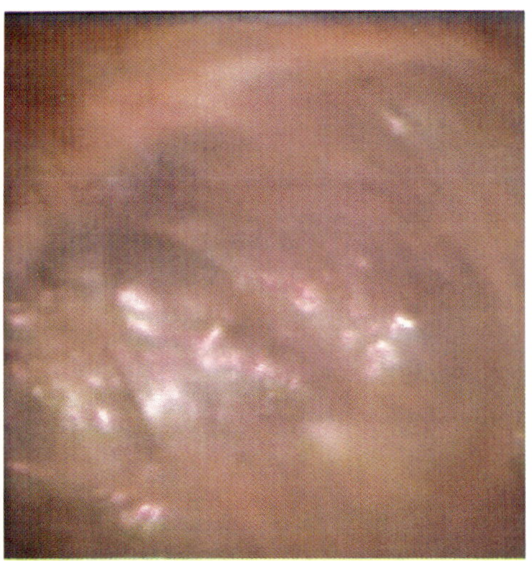

FIG. 13-26   A close-up of Fig. 13-25.

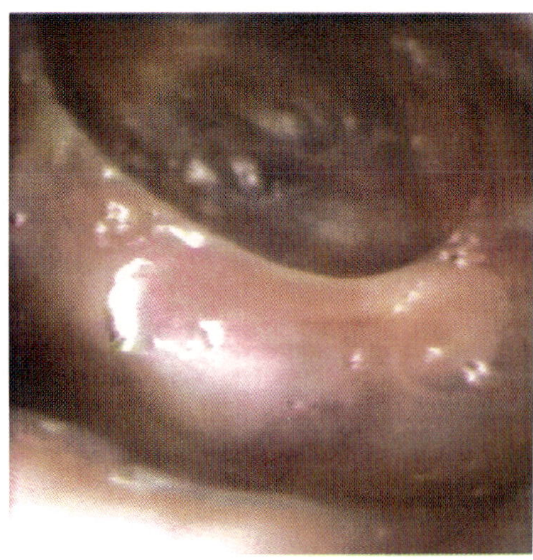

FIG. 13-27   Severe inflammation and luminal adhesions induced by uterine therapy.

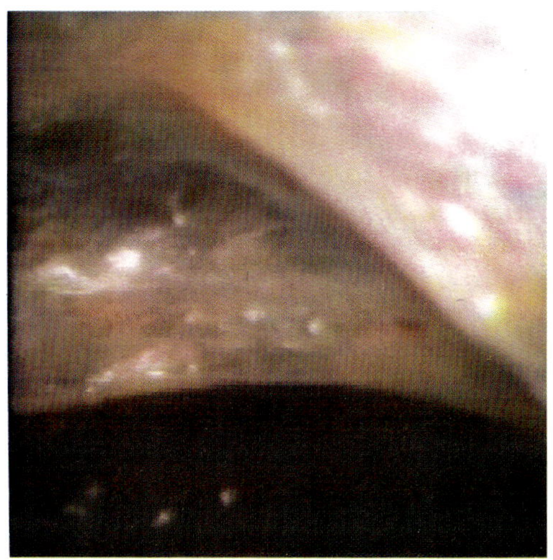

FIG. 13-28 Extensive adhesions of the uterine lumen following inappropriate therapy. What appears to be fluid resting dorsally is actually the web-like beginning of a thick, transluminal adhesion.

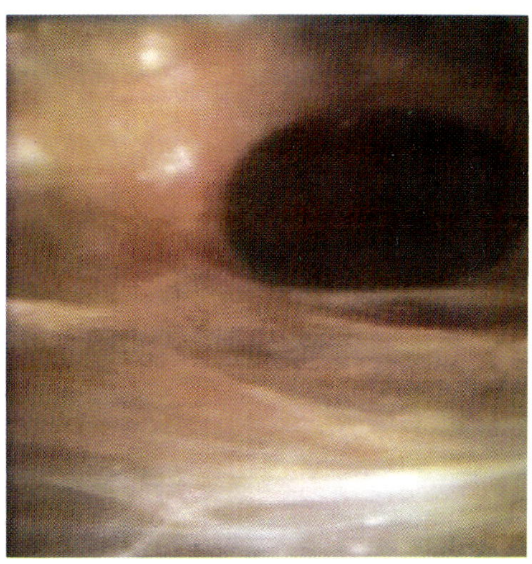

FIG. 13-29 Extensive scarring after infusion of an unknown substance.

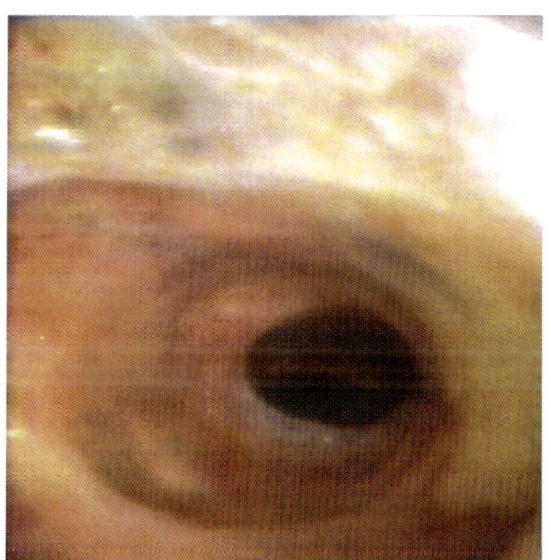

FIG. 13-30 Further into the uterine horn of the previous case (Fig. 13-29). The inflammatory response following inappropriate uterine therapy was pervasive throughout the uterine body and horns.

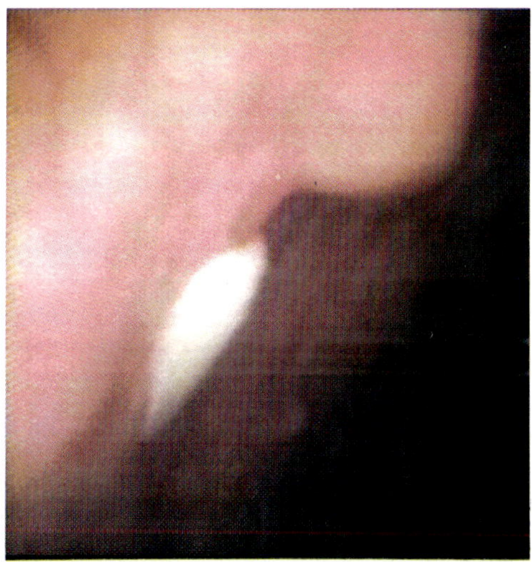

FIG. 13-31 Plaque attached to the endometrium. Uterine swabs revealed heavy growth of *Candida* sp.

REASONS AND JUSTIFICATION FOR ENDOSCOPY IN THE MARE

One must emphasize that this is not a procedure that is necessary for all broodmares. It is best utilized when all previously listed diagnostic tests have failed to determine the cause for the infertility or if a specific lesion exists. The technique is invasive and time-consuming, yet it may in many instances provide valuable information unavailable by any other route as well as the reason for the mare's infertility.

REFERENCES

1. Baker CB and Kenney RM: Systematic approach to the diagnosis of the infertile or subfertile mare. In Morrow DA, editor, Current therapy in theriogenology; diagnosis, treatment, and prevention of reproductive diseases in animals, Philadelphia, 1980, WB Saunders Co.
2. Blandy JP and Fowler CG: Lower tract endoscopy, Br Med Bull 42(3):280, 1986.
3. Devine DA and Lindsay FEF: Hysteroscopy in the cow using a flexible fiberscope, Vet Rec 115:627, 1984.
4. Grellner J: Equine endoscopy, Vet Technician 9(8):440, 1988.
5. Howard DJ and Lund VJ: Endoscopic surgery in otolaryngology, Br Med Bull 42(3):234, 1986.
6. Johnson JH et al: Selection and care of endoscopic equipment Proc AAEP, 239, 1977.
7. Miller RA: Endoscopic instrumentation: evolution, physical principles and clinical aspects, Br Med Bull 42(3):223, 1986.
8. Miller RA: Endoscopic surgery of the upper urinary tract, Br Med Bull, 42(3):274, 1986.
9. Muir WW and Robertson JT: Visceral analgesia: effects of xylazine, butorphanol, meperidine, and pentazocine in horses, AJVR 46(10):2081, 1985.
10. Pellicer A and Diamond MP: Distending media for hysteroscopy, Obstet Gynecol Clin North Am 15(1):23, 1988.
11. Shapiro BS: Instrumentation in hysteroscopy, Obst Gynec Clin North Am 15(1):13, 1988.
12. Sullins KE and Traub-Dargatz JL: Endoscopic anatomy of the equine urinary tract, Comp Cont Education 6(11):S663, 1984.
13. Valle RF: Future growth and development of hysteroscopy, Obstet Gynecol Clin North Am 15(1):111, 1988.
14. Weinberg JJ and Smith AD: Endourology and ureteroscopy Medical Instrumentation, 22(2):61, 1988.
15. Wilson AD and Ferguson JG: Use of a flexible fiberoptic laparoscope as a diagnostic aid in cattle, Canadian Vet J 25:229, 1984.
16. Wilson GL: Clinical experience with equine hysteroscopy. In Morrow DA, editor: Current therapy in theriogenology; diagnosis, treatment and prevention of reproductive diseases in small and large animals, ed 2, Philadelphia, 1986, WB Saunders Co.
17. Wilson GL: Hysteroscopic examination of mares, Veterinary Medicine/Small Animal Clinician 78:568, 1983.

Chapter 14

DIAGNOSTIC LAPAROSCOPY

A.T. FISCHER, JR.

Laparoscopy offers increased information regarding the abdominal cavity while being only slightly more invasive than percutaneous biopsy. With proper anatomic orientation and equipment, the dorsal abdominal cavity can be readily observed in the standing animal.

LAPAROSCOPIC TECHNIQUES
Equipment

The equipment employed in equine laparoscopy is the same as used in human laparoscopy and is available from many different manufacturers. Custom-built laparoscopes are also available in longer lengths and with different viewing angles. The laparoscopic cannula* is a sleeve through which the trocar, obturator, and telescope are inserted. Side ports for gas insufflation are desirable. Many different sizes for laparoscopes† exist. User preference dictates the size and view angle employed. Obviously, larger diameter laparoscopic telescopes are capable of transmitting more light, hence obtaining better views. Offset angles facilitate the viewing of

---

*Straight trocar and cannula with trumpet valve and oneway stopcock No. 57, Richard Wolf Medical Instruments Corp., Rosemont, Ill.
†Wolf Lumina 130 degree No. 51250, Wolf Lumina 170 degree type 4938.31 No. 122504, Richard Wolf Medical Instruments Corp., Rosemont, Ill.

objects that are difficult to visualize with the straight-ahead viewing telescopes. Operating laparoscopes allow the insertion of an instrument parallel with the telescope, ensuring accurate instrument placement.

The power (wattage) of the light source is important; mainly if one wishes to use videotape or take photographs. Viewing structures directly through the laparoscope requires only a 150-watt light source. Video and photographic setups require from 300 to 1000 watts. Special flash generators are available for photography.

Insufflation of the abdomen is provided by carbon dioxide or nitrogen sources with a pressure and flow regulator.* Alternatively, we have used the exhaust from a suction apparatus with a bacterial filter with no untoward effects.

Probes to manipulate or biopsy viscera are useful. These probes are introduced through a second puncture site and may be inserted through a cannula. We currently use uterine biopsy forceps to perform biopsies and move structures. Further manipulation of viscera may be obtained by an assistant palpating per rectum.

Patient preparation

The animal should be fasted for 18 to 24 hours before laparoscopic examination of the abdomen, unless an emergency situation exists. It is not necessary or desirable to withhold water. The animal is restrained in standing stocks with the tail tied to prevent it from contaminating the surgical field. Abdominal palpation per rectum should precede laparoscopy to ensure that there are no adherent masses in the area selected for insertion of the laparoscope. Both paralumbar fossae are prepared for aseptic surgery. The animal is administered a sedative analgesic combination (e.g., xylazine 0.44 mg/kg and butorphanol tartrate 0.022 mg/kg) before the start of the procedure. Broad spectrum perioperative antibiotics may be administered if desired.

Technique

After suitable sedation has been achieved, adherent draping material† is placed over the paralumbar fossa. Local anesthetic agents are infused subcutaneously and intramuscularly into the sites selected for the insertion of the laparoscopic cannula and instruments. The most common site of insertion is at the dorsal edge of the crus of the internal abdominal oblique muscle midway between the tuber coxae and the ribs. Using the middle of the paralumbar fossa facilitates examination both cranially and caudally. It is impor-

---

*Wolf automatic CO_2 insufflator, type 569, Richard Wolf Medical Instruments Corp., Rosemont, Ill.
†Steridrape 1050, 3M, St. Paul, Minn.

tant not to go too far dorsally in the paralumbar fossa, or retroperitoneal insertion of the laparoscope may occur with subsequent damage to the kidney. Shortly coupled horses (i.e., horses with a small space between the last rib and the tuber coxa) can be difficult to examine because the laparoscope will have limited mobility. In these patients, selection of laparoscopes with angled lenses is appropriate.

Having achieved local anesthesia of the insertion sites, a skin incision is made to allow the laparoscopic cannula and trocar to be inserted. Insufflation of the abdomen with a Verres needle will facilitate introduction of the laparoscope in patients with large amounts of fat. In the average horse this has not been necessary. The laparoscopic cannula, with its sharp trocar, is inserted through the muscle layers into the abdomen. (We have modified a trocar by blunting the sharp tip for the final penetration into the abdominal cavity. The use of the dull obturator minimizes the chance of viscus penetration but increases the difficulty in penetrating the peritoneum.)

Following entrance into the abdominal cavity, insufflation is started by using carbon dioxide or other filtered gas. Units available commercially with pressure and flow controls may be employed. Abdominal distention pressures in the range of 20 cm water are necessary to maximize visualization of structures. The telescope is inserted through the cannula and examination of the dorsal abdominal cavity is performed.

The laparoscopic telescope is removed from the cannula and the insufflating gas allowed to escape once the procedure is considered completed. Should examination of the contralateral side be desired, the laparoscopic procedure should be repeated on the opposite side before allowing the insufflating gas to escape. In most cases, I routinely examine both sides of the abdomen.

At the end of the procedure, the insufflating gas is allowed to escape and skin sutures are placed. It is normal for there to be mild subcutaneous emphysema after surgery, but this has not been a problem. The subcutaneous emphysema may be minimized by allowing the insufflating gas to escape and by not suturing the first skin incision until both sides have been examined. Mild colic signs may be noticed if excessive amounts of insufflating gas remain.

NORMAL ANATOMY

Left side

The laparoscope is inserted into the left paralumbar fossa in the region of the nephrosplenic ligament (Figs. 14-1 to 14-11). It is probably safer to direct the laparoscope caudally during insertion to minimize trauma to the spleen. Puncture of the spleen has occurred

Text continued on p. 179.

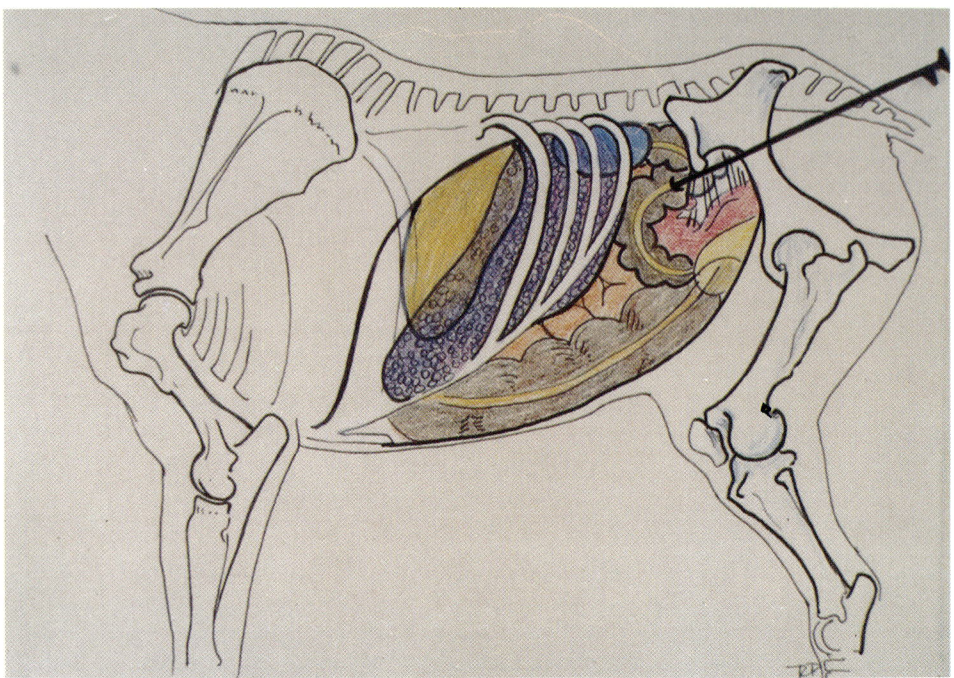

FIG. 14-1 Insertion site for laparoscope on left side of horse.

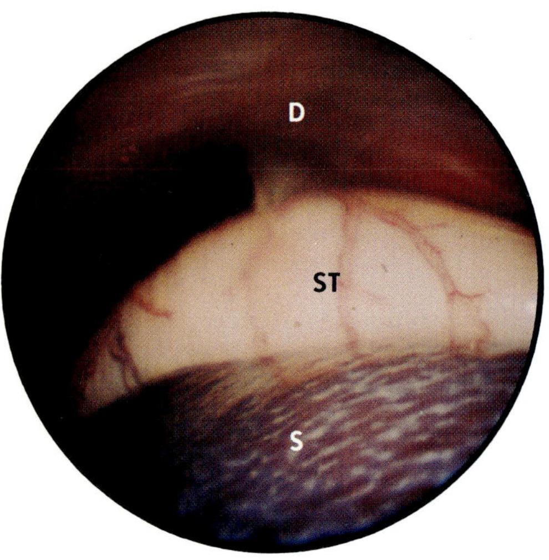

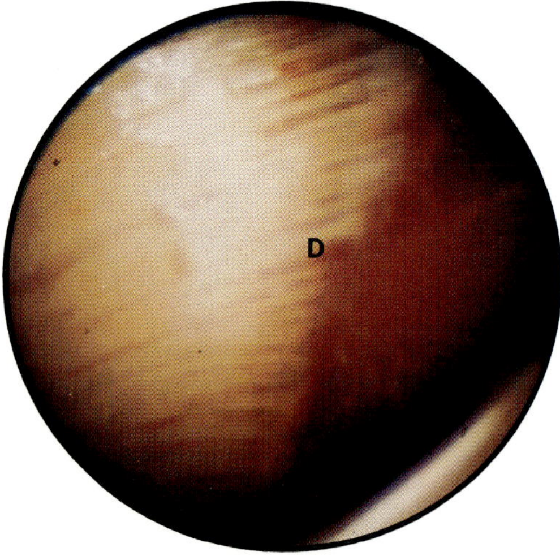

FIG. 14-2 Laparoscopic view of rostral left abdomen. Diaphragm (D), stomach (ST), spleen (S).

FIG. 14-3 Laparoscopic view of rostral left abdomen. Close-up view of diaphragm *(D)* at musculotendinous junction.

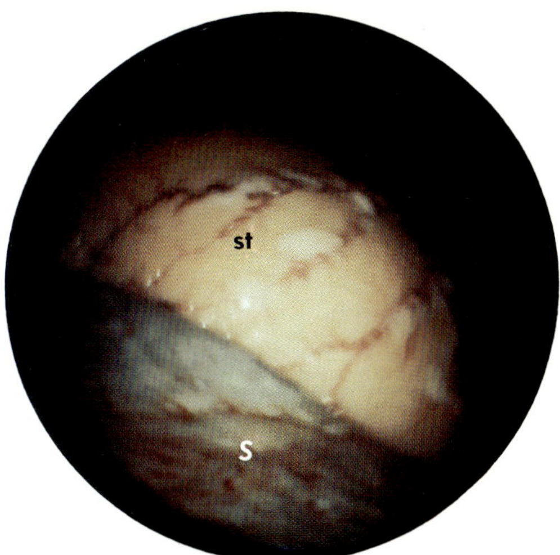

FIG. 14-4   **Laparoscopic view of rostral left abdomen.** Spleen (s) and stomach (St). Note fibrin tags on the stomach.

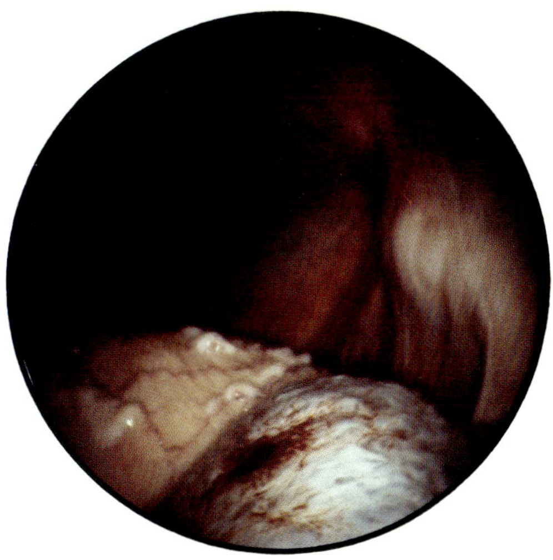

FIG. 14-5   **Laparoscopic view of rostral left abdomen.** Fibrin tags on stomach, hemorrhage from splenic biopsy site.

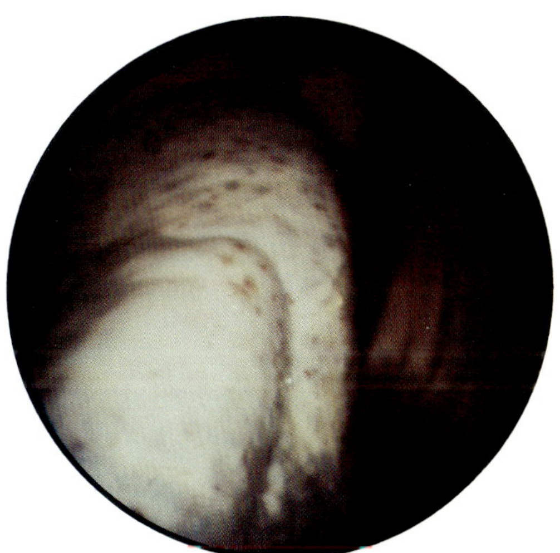

FIG. 14-6   **Laparoscopic view of rostral left abdomen.** Spleen and nephrosplenic ligament.

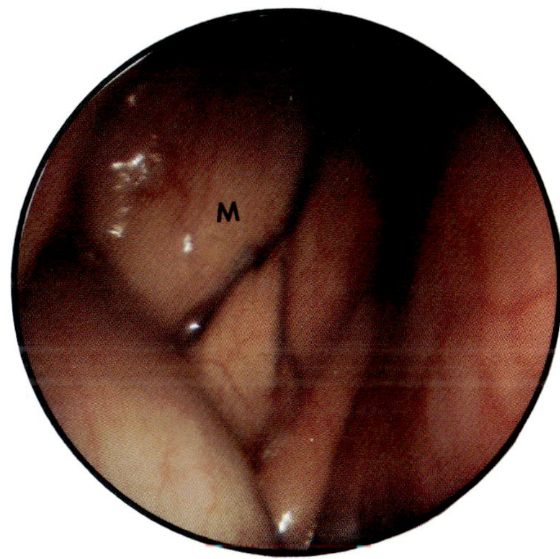

FIG. 14-7   **Laparoscopic view of middle left abdomen.** Sheet of mesentery *(M)* and small intestine in foreground.

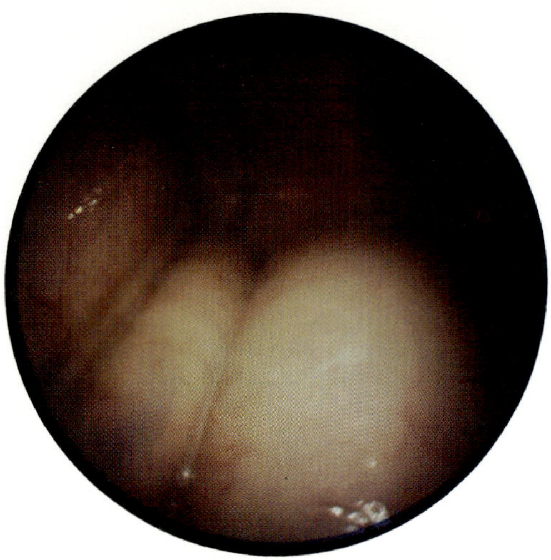

FIG. 14-8   Laparoscopic view of mid left abdomen. Small intestine.

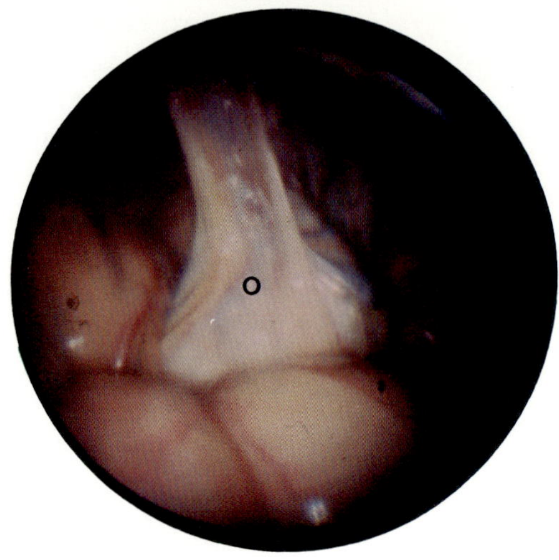

FIG. 14-9   Laparoscopic view of mid left abdomen. Ovary *(O)*.

(Reprinted with permission from Fischer Jr AT: J Am Vet Med Assoc 189:289, 1986.)

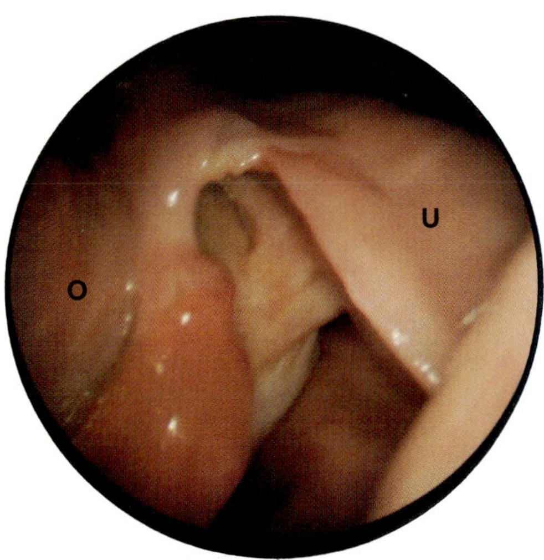

FIG. 14-10   Laparoscopic view of mid left abdomen. Ovary *(O)* and uterus *(U)*.

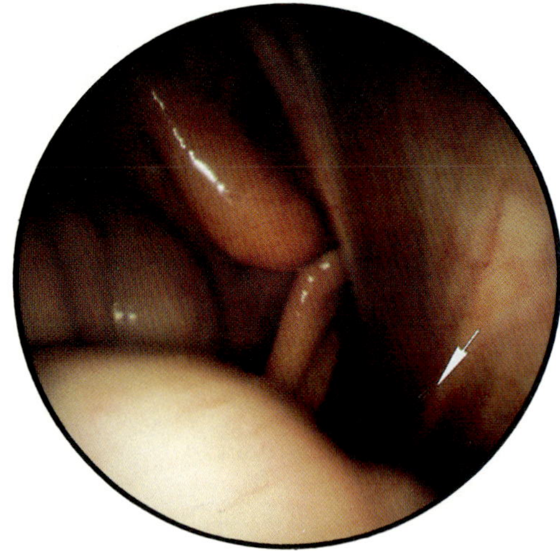

FIG. 14-11   Laparoscopic view of caudal left abdomen. Arrow points at inguinal ring.

during laparoscope insertion and has not been associated with excessive hemorrhage but obviously should be avoided. When viewing caudally, the urogenital tract will be apparent. In the female, the ovary hangs from the broad ligament. The ovary is connected to the uterus by the proper ligament of the ovary. The infundibulum may be seen. The uterine horn can be followed caudally to the body. Dorsal to the uterus, the descending small colon is evident and easily identified if a palpators hand is introduced per rectum. Below the uterus, the urinary bladder is evident. Looking laterally towards the left body wall, the inguinal ring can be observed. In the female, the blood vessels, nerves, and lymphatics coursing through the ring may be observed. In the male, the ductus deferens and the testicular vessels can be seen on their way to the ampulla of the ductus deferens. A cryptorchid testicle may be seen in this area.

As the laparoscope is directed straight into the abdomen, the mesenteric root can be seen. Isolated parts of the small and large intestine will also be seen. Currently, it is not possible to follow the small and large intestine systematically using the laparoscope. The fat surrounding the left kidney can be seen by looking rostrally from the ovary. The spleen and nephrosplenic ligament can be observed by looking farther forward. By looking over the nephrosplenic ligament, the dorsal aspect of the stomach is evident. The diaphragm is seen rostral and lateral to the stomach. Occasionally, the left lateral lobe of the liver may be evident on this side.

Right side

Many of the structures seen on the left side will also be evident on the right side (Figs. 14-12 to 14-15). By starting the examination caudally, the urogenital structures will be seen. When looking into the middle of the abdominal cavity, the small colon and small intestine will be evident. Slightly rostral to this, the attachment of the cecum to the dorsal body wall will be evident. The descending duodenum is seen here as it goes around the root of the mesentery. It may be followed orally on the right or lateral side of the root of the mesentery. The large colon and cecum can be visualized in part by looking ventrally and forward. The right lobe of the liver may be viewed dorsally and can be easily biopsied by inserting a biopsy forceps through the paralumbar fossa. The right kidney is not particularly evident because of its retroperitoneal location.

Ventrally located structures may be examined by positioning the animal in dorsal recumbency, under general anesthesia, and inserting the laparoscope through the linea alba.

Indications for Laparoscopy

CONDITION OR AREA	FIGURE
Abdominal tumor	(Fig. 14-16)
Abdominal abscess	(Fig. 14-21)
Examination of the dorsal aspect of the stomach	
Liver biopsy and examination of portions of the liver	
Spleen biopsy and examination of portions of the spleen	
Kidney biopsy and examination of kidneys	(Fig. 14-19)
Ovarian and urogenital tract examination	
Location of cryptorchid testicles	
Evaluation of peritonitis	(Fig. 14-20)
Evaluation of rectal tears	
Evaluation of the abdominal cavity for metastatic disease	
Evaluation of abnormal rectal palpation	
Evaluation of chronic colic	

Text continued on p. 184.

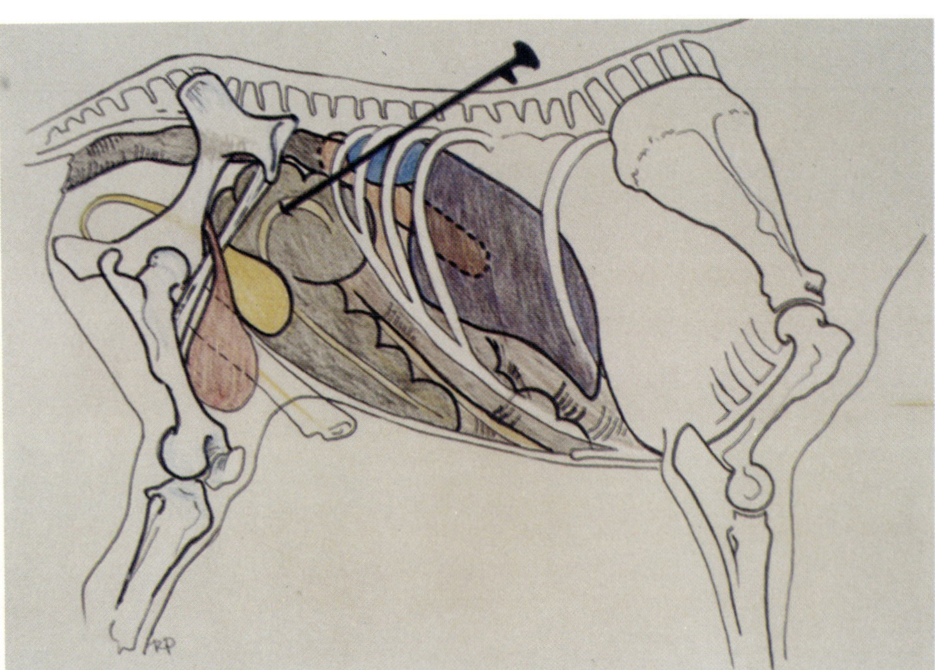

FIG. 14-12 Insertion site for laparoscope on the right side of the abdomen.

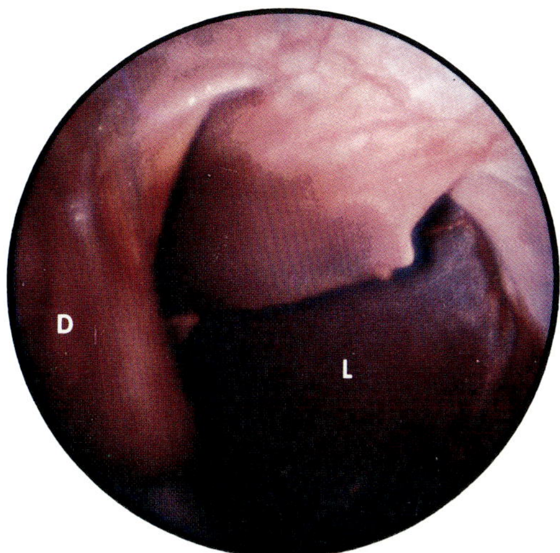

FIG. 14-13   Laparoscopic view of rostral right abdomen. Descending duodenum *(D)* and liver *(L)*.

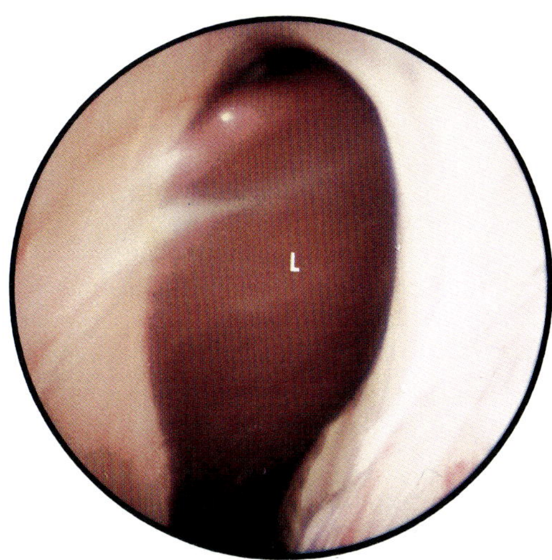

FIG. 14-14   Laparoscopic view of rostral right abdomen. Close-up view of liver *(L)*.

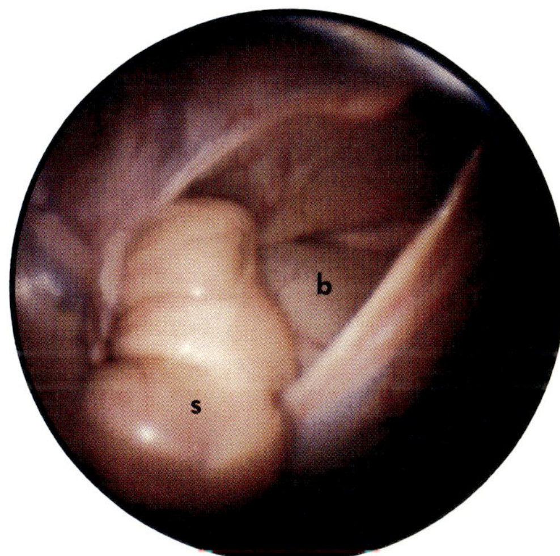

FIG. 14-15   Laparoscopic view of caudal right abdomen. Small colon *(S)* and urinary bladder *(b)*.

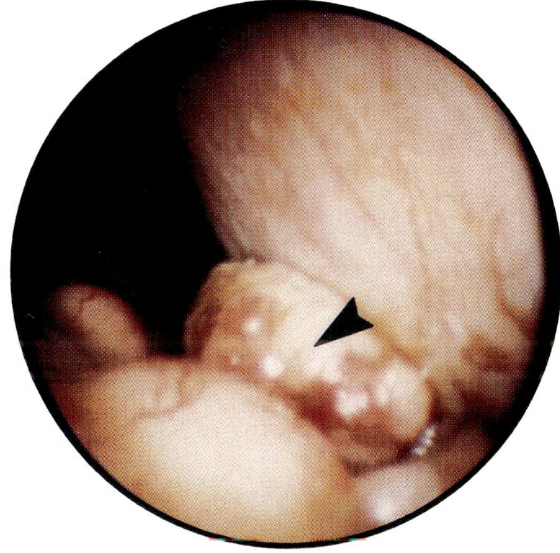

FIG. 14-16   Metastatic nodule from ovarian teratoma *(arrow)* on nephrosplenic ligament.

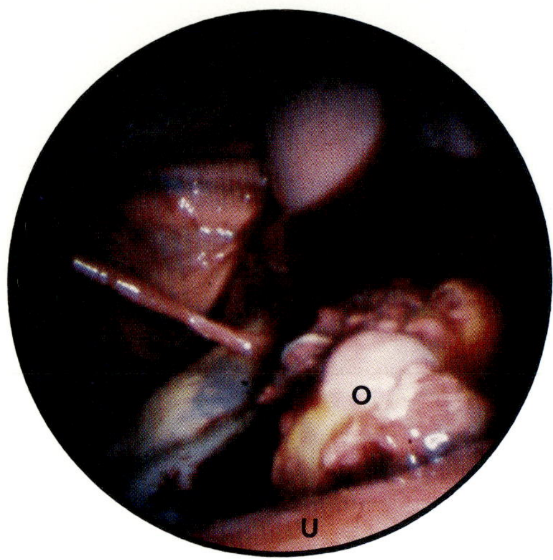

FIG. 14-17   Ovarian teratoma *(O)*
adjacent to uterus *(u)*. Note
hemorrhagic peritoneal fluid.

(Reprinted with permission from Fischer Jr AT:
J Am Vet Med Assoc 189:289, 1986.)

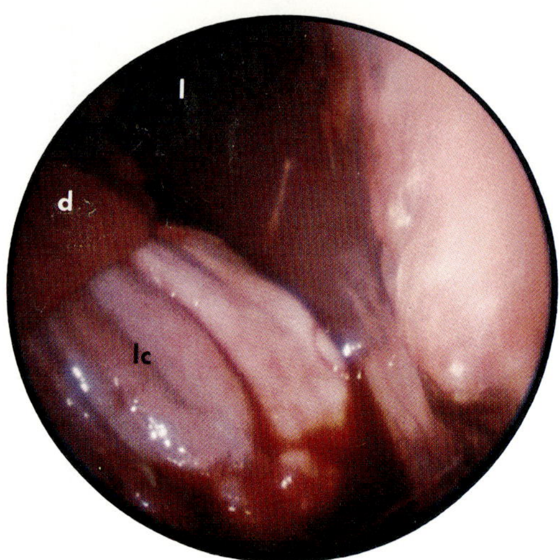

FIG. 14-18   Descending duodenum
(d), cecum *(lc)*, and liver *(l)*. Note
increased hemorrhagic peritoneal fluid
secondary to ovarian teratoma.

(Reprinted with permission from Fischer Jr AT:
J Am Vet Med Assoc 189:289, 1986.)

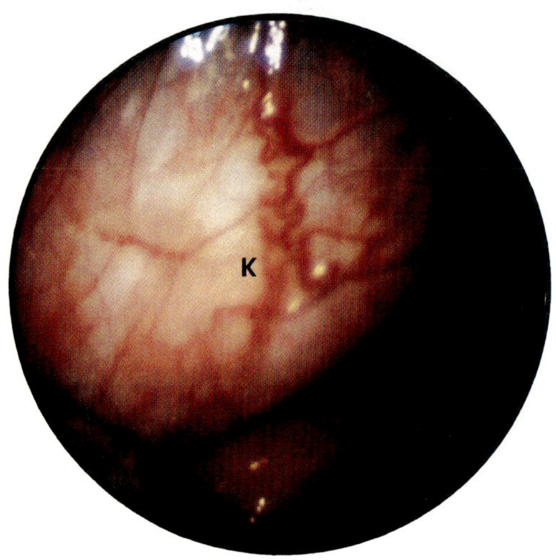

FIG. 14-19   Enlarged left kidney *(k)*
secondary to ureteral calculi.

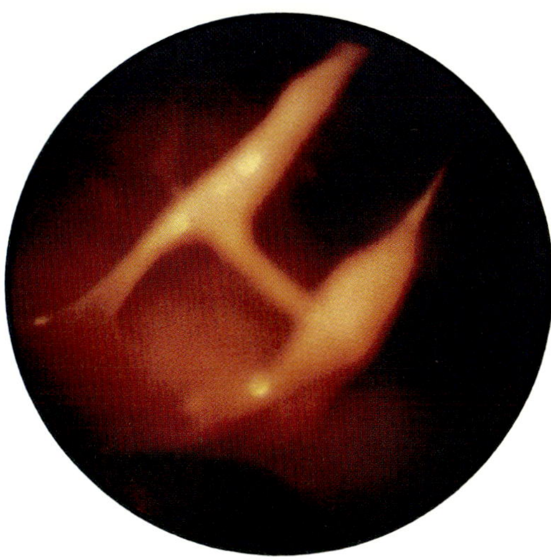

FIG. 14-20 Fibrin tags associated with fibrinous peritonitis.

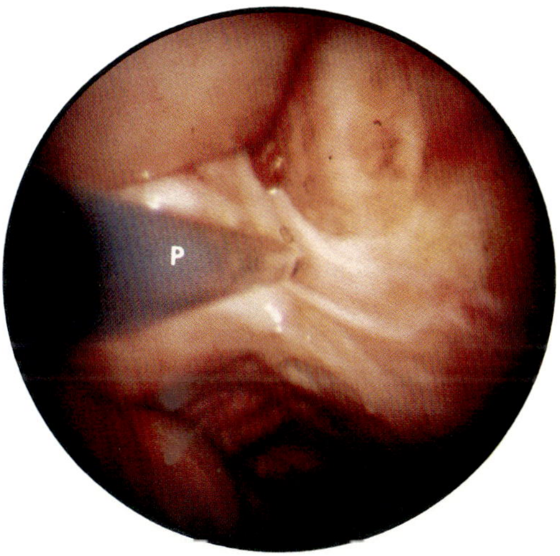

FIG. 14-21 Adhesion between abdominal abscess and uterus. Probe *(P)* is on adhesion.

(Reprinted with permission from Fischer Jr AT: J Am Vet Med Assoc 189:289, 1986.)

COMPLICATIONS

Complications are seldom encountered if the laparoscope is inserted properly. As mentioned previously, trauma to the spleen and kidney may occur on the left side of the abdominal cavity. Hemorrhage that has occurred in these instances has been minor. Perforation of the cecum may occur when inserting the laparoscope on the right side if care is not exercised or if the animal's cecum is greatly distended. Subcutaneous emphysema will occur routinely, but has not caused any clinical problems. Only partial thickness biopsies (serosal surface) should be performed only on gastrointestinal or other hollow organs. The liver and spleen can be safely biopsied. It should be remembered, if one intends to examine serial abdominocentesis samples, that laparoscopy is associated with an increase in abdominal white blood cell counts and peritoneal protein.

Contraindications to laparoscopy include diaphragmatic hernia and obstructive bowel disease with distended viscus such as the large intestine.

BIBLIOGRAPHY

Fischer AT et al: Diagnostic laparoscopy in the horse, J Am Vet Med Assoc 189:289, 1986.

Witherspoon DM, Kraemer DC, and Seager SW: Laparoscopy in the horse. In Harrison RM and Wildt DE, editors: Animal laparoscopy, Baltimore, 1980, Williams & Wilkins Co.

INDEX